Healthy Hearts, Healthy Women

How Women Can Prevent or Reverse Heart Disease

Christine L. Wells, Ph.D., FACSM

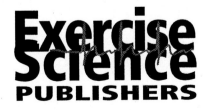

Exercise Science PUBLISHERS

Exercise Science Publishers

Layout and cover design: Paul Lewis

Library of Congress Number: 2001087606

ISBN: 1-58518-412-8

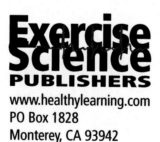

Exercise Science PUBLISHERS
www.healthylearning.com
PO Box 1828
Monterey, CA 93942

FOR ALL WOMEN—EVERYWHERE.

And their children, husbands, lovers, and friends.

ACKNOWLEDGMENTS

My acknowledgments list is short, but of no less importance than if it went on for pages. After a long career as a university professor I must thank my students for all the questions they asked. It was my continual seeking for answers to those questions that kept me up-to-date on the literature.

And it was my working experiences with women that gave me the encouragement I needed to believe that I had something to offer them about everyday, but important, health issues. My thanks to these women. May this book (as well as others to follow) empower them to take control of their lives and health.

I had the help of an editor, Fran Mummings. She kept me on target and offered lots of encouragement when my resolve faded. She also made the copy editor's job far easier. My thanks, too, to Dr. Barbara Drinkwater, who got me into this in the first place, and to Dr. Rick Frey, for his encouragement, enthusiasm, and occasional hand holding. They are wonderful colleagues to have in your corner. And finally, my thanks to Anita Hopkins. She kept hot meals on the table, and our two cats company during the late hours that are my working style.

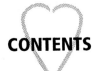

CONTENTS

CONTENTS
continued

Introduction to Part I:
A Woman's Heart

It is tragic that women's heart disease has been so long ignored. How many people are aware that more women die from heart disease than men? Not many. Unfortunately, most research on cardiovascular disease has been completed in men. Thus I had relatively little information to reply on as I developed the material for this book. Although the basic risk factors for heart disease seem to be universal, most people remain totally uninformed about these risk factors in women. Further, there are definite differences between men and women relative to the *prevalence* of a risk factor, and/or the *magnitude of its effect*. These differences are quite important, and that's the reason this book is needed.

Some are inclined to believe that heart disease—is heart disease. But the differences between men and women should not be downplayed. It is quite obvious that women haven't benefited as much as men from the wealth of knowledge that is available on diseases of the heart and blood vessels, and I believe there are two reasons for this. One is that women are not particularly well informed about heart disease—except as it relates to the men in their lives. They are certainly NOT well informed about heart disease in themselves—probably because most believe it is primarily "a man's disease." The second reason is that many physicians are not particularly well informed either, and so women don't get the attention they should get when it comes to examining them for heart disease early in life.

The good news is that research is currently underway, through the Women's Health Initiative, to expand our knowledge about heart disease in women. While we wait for that "new" information to come forth—and it will take another ten years and maybe more for it to be disseminated widely—we need to recognize what is currently known, and use it to our fullest advantage. We can't wait—too many women are dying—now. That's why this book was written.

THE PURPOSES OF THIS BOOK

There are four primary goals or purposes of this book.

- ❤ FIRST: to convince you that the dangers of heart and vascular disease are very real and important health problems for women.

- ❤ SECOND: to enable you to evaluate your individual and unique risks, for diseases of the heart and blood vessels.

- ❤ THIRD: to inspire and empower you to control your heart-health—both mentally and physically. This is something you CAN do something about, you just need the desire and the will to do so.

- ❤ FOURTH: to provide the means—the "how-to"—by which you can alter your lifestyle to one that is heart-healthy with aerobic exercise, a non-atherogenic diet, and a life of lovingkindness to yourself and others.

WHO IS THIS BOOK FOR?

This book is written first of all for women who are "at risk" for diseases of the heart and blood vessels. In some cases you know who you are. You know that you have one or more of the major cardiovascular risk factors because someone has told you so or because you read about it. In other cases, you do not yet know whether you are "at risk" for heart disease. When you read Chapter 3 you will think that all women are at risk, and in a sense, that is potentially true. In Chapter 4 you will find out whether or not *you* are truly at risk or not. If you are, then your focus will be on *primary prevention*, which means preventing the initial development of heart or blood vessel disease.

This book is also for any woman who currently has heart disease. Although coronary heart disease will be more fully defined and described in the next chapter, YOU know who you are. If a doctor has ever told you you have hypertension, heart disease or blood vessel disease, or you have been under treatment for any of these diseases, then you *must* read this book. Perhaps your doctor has recommended you read it to begin *secondary prevention*. What we are preventing in this instance is, quite frankly, a heart attack or a *second* heart attack, in a person who already has vascular disease. Of course, you need to do more than "read" the book. But I'm getting ahead of myself. Suffice to say right now—this book is for you.

The book should also be read by anyone who has a loved one "at risk" or already diagnosed with heart disease. This means husbands, lovers, companions, cohabitants, significant others—whatever the label! It also means mothers and daughters. So pass it around. The more you know about heart disease, the better. The more you know, the more supportive and understanding you will be of people who have heart disease. The more you know, the healthier we will all be.

WHAT'S TO COME IN PART I: A WOMAN'S HEART

Part I consists of Chapters 1 through 5. You'll learn quite a lot about heart disease and its risk factors, with particular emphasis on how this information pertains to women.

Chapter 1, *Do Women Get Heart Disease?* sets the record straight about the incidence (rate of new cases) and prevalence (number of existing cases) of heart disease in women. Most likely you will be shocked. Heart disease is the number one killer of American women, and the death rate is NOT declining as it is in men.

Chapter 2, *Understanding Heart Disease* will tell you exactly what heart disease is, how it develops, its signs and symptoms, and the medical conditions that result. Consider this chapter a primer on heart disease in women, because, that's exactly what it is.

Chapter 3, *Who Is at Risk*, is long—not only because there are many risk factors to consider, but because some affect women differently than men. Many of these risk factors are highly related to one another, and this is particularly so in women. You'll learn about the metabolic syndrome and why it is so important to see that all the variables are associated with one another.

Chapter 4, *Your Heart Disease Risk Profile*, will enable you to specifically determine YOUR risk for heart disease. It provides a series of "profiles" that allow you to estimate your risk for each of the major risk factors recognized for women. This chapter is quite unique among other books written on heart disease, because you can rate yourself on each risk factor to develop a comprehensive personal risk profile. This chapter, of course, is directed primarily to those readers who do not currently have heart disease— or at least—are not yet aware they have it.

Chapter 5, *Estrogen and Heart Disease: What's the Connection?*, is also a unique chapter. It addresses the connection between estrogen—the hormone that truly makes a woman, a woman—and heart disease. The good news is that estrogen may protect women from heart disease—at least in early life, but the bad news is that we have menopause, and our estrogen levels decline significantly. Along with that loss, we lose our cardio-protection. It is because of this that considerable attention is given to menopausal estrogen therapy—its possible benefits to our heart and bone health, and its possible risks relative to endometrial and breast cancer. It is very important that every woman evaluate this issue—perhaps with the assistance of a physician—relative to her own health needs and characteristics, and not simply decide for or against taking estrogen on the basis of heresy or general information.

Part II of this book deals with what you—personally—can do about all this. **Chapters 7, 8 and 9** describe a lifestyle program that will *prevent* heart disease in those currently free of symptoms, and that will *reverse* atherosclerosis in those who currently have heart disease.

You may be so anxious to begin this lifestyle program, that you'll want to read Part II either before or in conjunction with Part I. If that is your wish, I recommend you begin with **Chapter 6**, *Change: Making the Commitment,* that deals with making a commitment to change while you also read Chapter 1. Whatever your style of reading a book, find yourself a secluded spot—perhaps with a pen or felt-tipped highlighter in hand, and read the entire book. It may save your life.

CHAPTER 1

Do Women Get Heart Disease?

> **"Heart disease is an equal opportunity killer."**
> **—Nanette Wenger, M.D.**

This may be the most important book you've ever read. Why? Because heart disease kills more women than any other cause of death. What you read here could save your life or the life of a loved one.

When most of us think about heart disease, we think (and worry) about our fathers or husbands, our uncles, and our brothers. That's because we've learned that heart disease is a man's disease, that women only rarely get heart disease. How wrong we are! And millions like us as well. Even many doctors are not fully informed.

THE NUMBER ONE CAUSE OF DEATH

Cardiovascular disease is an all inclusive term used for diseases of the heart, the arteries and the veins. Taken all together, cardiovascular diseases are the number one cause of death—all ages, all persons—in the United States. In fact, cardiovascular diseases cause about as many deaths each year as the next eight leading causes of death combined. The most common form of cardiovascular disease is *coronary heart disease*. Sometimes called *CHD*, I will most often refer to coronary heart disease simply as "heart disease." Heart disease occurs when disease affects the major arteries of the heart—the coronary arteries—so heart disease is coronary vascular disease.

This book is specifically about heart disease in women. How it develops, what symptoms result, and what you can do to prevent it or reverse it. To set the record straight about women and heart disease, let's look at some statistics culled from the latest data from the American Heart Association and the Centers for Disease Control and Prevention.

HEART DISEASE IN WOMEN

A great deal of publicity has informed us that death rates from heart and vascular diseases have declined in the last several decades. Of course, that's good news. What is less well known is that the rate of decline is far less in women than in men, and even less in minority women than in white women.

No one can dispute that our population is growing older; the "greying" of America is well documented. About 34 million Americans are currently over the age of 65, and the majority are women. This is important because about 84% of all heart disease deaths occur in people over the age of 65.

Not only is our population getting older, it is increasing in size. So even while the overall death rate is decreasing, the absolute number of deaths due to diseases of the heart in women is increasing. Since 1984, the number of deaths from cardiovascular disease in women has *exceeded* the number in men. In 1995, the most recent year for which there is complete data, the total number of deaths in women from these diseases was 505,440. It was (only!) 455,152 in men. Heart and blood vessel disease kills more women in the US than all forms of cancer, lung disease, pneumonia, diabetes, accidents and AIDS *combined*.

But I don't want to give you the notion that heart disease is only a disease of elderly women. The 76 million "baby boomers" are persons born after World War II between the years 1946 and 1964. That currently puts them in the 35 to 44 and the 45 to 54 year age groups (groups used for government statistics). In 1993, the death rate from diseases of the heart for women in the 35 to 44 age group was 18.6 (per 100,000) for white women and 70.2 (!) for black women. In the 45 to 54 year old group, these death rates were 63.6 for white women and 206.0 for black women (all rates are expressed per 100,000 population). Note the sharp increase with age, and the rather extreme difference between white and black women. And heart disease is more common in Hispanic women too. The Corpus Christi Heart Project revealed not only higher rates for heart attack in Mexican-American women than non-Hispanic white women, but also higher fatalities. These numbers are far from trivial—and they indicate considerable disparity among ethnic groups. Most importantly, they clearly indicate that "young" women get heart disease—and that many die from it.

Heart attack and other diseases of the heart and blood vessels are the number one killers of American women over age 35.

Of course, not everyone with heart disease dies from it—at least not at first. An estimated 1 in every 5 American women currently has some form of heart or vascular disease. This is referred to as *prevalence*—the extent of existing cases. Clearly heart disease is not just a disease that men get. Heart disease is as much a woman's disease as a man's disease. As one famous (woman) cardiologist has stated, "Heart disease is an equal opportunity killer."

HEART ATTACK

A frequent manifestation of heart disease is "heart attack." Heart attack—two words that strike nearly paralyzing fear in anyone—may be fatal or nonfatal.

Heart attack is the single largest killer of American women. In 1993, it claimed the lives of 239,701 women, 48.9% of all cardiovascular deaths. Fatal heart attack and fatal cardiac arrest constitute *sudden death* (unexpected death that occurs almost immediately after the onset of symptoms). Of considerable concern is the fact that nearly two-thirds of all sudden death in women occurs with no previous symptoms or warnings. And, once again, heart attack does *not* just occur in the elderly. In 35 to 44 year old women, heart disease death rates are 27.1 (per 100,000) for white women and 65.4 for black women. About 19,990 women under the age of 65 die of heart attack each year. More than 31% of these, are under the age of 55! But not every woman who has a heart attack dies from it. In fact, over 6,800,000 women who are alive today have had a heart attack, angina (chest pain), or both. In 1995 alone, 858,000 women diagnosed with coronary heart disease were released from hospitals.

In addition, a woman's prospects for a lasting return to a normal life following a heart attack are far gloomier than a man's. Forty-four percent of women who have heart attacks will die within the first year compared to 27% of men. Recurrence is also more likely in women. During the first six years after a heart attack, 31% of women will have a second attack compared with 23% of men; about 20% will be disabled with congestive heart failure, and about 34% will develop angina. At older ages, women who have heart attacks are more likely than men to die from them within a few weeks.

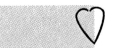

Heart attack is the single largest killer of American women. 44% of women who have a heart attack will die within 1 year. More than 6,800,000 women who are alive today have had a heart attack, angina or both.

A WOMAN'S RISK

Taken all together, almost half of all women in the United States will die of heart or vascular disease. According to the American Heart Association, one in nine women in the 45 to 64 age group has some form of heart or blood vessel disease. This risk soars to one in three after age 65.

It is obviously a myth that heart disease is a man's disease.

It is a myth that heart disease is a man's disease. Heart disease is the number one killer of American women.

WHY DOES THIS MYTH EXIST?

Why is heart disease ignored in women? Why does this myth—that heart disease in women is of minor significance—exist? The most logical reason is that men are generally affected at a much earlier age than women—by about 10 years. Thus, the death rate from heart disease for men at age 40 is not attained by women until after age 50. When a large number of men are struck down "in the prime of life"—that gets attention. And many of these deaths are from "sudden death"—which is particularly dramatic because it is so unexpected—and catastrophic.

It's true—when matched for age—women have less *atherosclerosis*, the thickening and hardening of artery walls that is the major cause of heart disease (and stroke), than men. The age-specific death rates from diseases of the heart are *much higher* before age 50 in men than in women. The male-to-female ratio of cardiac-related deaths from age 35 to about 50 is almost 6 to 1. That's why *nearly all the research* on cardiovascular disease, and particularly coronary heart disease—has been done on men. At least that's the usual reason given. There may be additional "socio-political" reasons I'll not discuss here but leave for your own speculation. The fact remains that practically all we know about heart disease comes from research completed with men as subjects. And, of course, that makes some sense. If you want to learn as much about heart disease as possible, study the group in which it is most prevalent.

But is it valid to assume that the results of these studies apply equally to women? That will probably remain a hot topic of discussion for quite some time, but fortunately, we have learned some things about women through the still ongoing Framingham Heart Study that began in the 50s, and the Nurses' Health Study, another ongoing study, that began in the 70s. In general, we've learned that most of the risk factors identified in men *generally* apply to women—only the *magnitude* of their effects may be different. This topic will be covered in Chapter 3.

Some important questions are: Why are young men more susceptible to heart disease than young women? and What, if any, gender-related factors offer a woman—a young woman, anyway—protection? Is there such a thing as "gender protection" from heart disease? There are no firm answers to these questions—yet. But we've learned a few things. For example, we know that long-term elevation in blood pressure (*hypertension*), although very common in women, is less predictive of heart attack than in men. We also know that *blood lipid profiles* (cholesterol and blood fat levels) in premenopausal women are more "cardio-protective" than in men, and the usual reason given for this is—you guessed it—estrogen. We also know that as men gain weight they add excess body fat in their abdominal region, a particularly dangerous risk factor for hypertension, elevated cholesterol, and heart disease. As women gain weight, extra fat is more typically placed on the hips and buttocks (bet you never thought that was "cardio-protective"). You'll learn more about these issues later in this book. We've also discovered that there are some "women-specific" risk factors for heart disease. The use of oral contraceptives may be one, and early hysterectomy another. Many believe that menopause—because it signals a sharp decline in the production of estrogen—is the worst risk factor of all for heart disease. I will explain why I don't believe this is so in Chapters 3 and 5.

IS THERE HARM IN THE MYTH?

Is there any danger in the myth—that women don't get heart disease? I believe there is. Such a misconception does not serve women well—and certainly does not serve YOU well. A healthcare provider who is not aware of the high rate of cardiovascular disease in women will not be alert to the symptoms of the disease in you. In fact, a nationwide Gallup poll recently found that nearly two-thirds of primary-care physicians were *not* aware that the symptoms of heart disease may be different in a woman than in a man. Physicians typically look for *angina*, which is classically described in men as crushing pain that begins in the chest and extends down the left arm and up into the jaw. But in women, symptoms may be simply short-ness of breath with or without exertion, and sometimes extreme fatigue and nausea. Angina in women may be little more than a tightening in the chest, and is often mistaken by doctors for heartburn, indigestion, or the symptoms of *hiatal hernia* (a condition causing regurgitation of acidic stom-ach contents into the esophagus). In fact, upper abdominal pain is a com-mon symptom in women who are having a heart attack, and consequently, heart attack may not be diagnosed until an electrocardiogram is com-pleted along with blood enzyme tests (both described in Chapter 3). If physicians were more aware—if women themselves were more aware—there would be fewer unnecessary delays in treatment, fewer initially mis-taken or delayed diagnoses, and many fatal *second* heart attacks could be prevented.

The existence of the myth may also cause women to neglect lower-ing their risk factors for heart disease because these risk factors simply do not seem important. Women may ignore symptoms that should be urgently treated—such as shortness of breath, or feelings of pressure in the chest. Symptoms that a woman may attribute to heartburn, or stress or depres-sion may, in reality, be early symptoms of coronary vascular disease.

Another danger of the myth is that when women do enter the medi-cal system, they may be treated less aggressively than men. For example, research has shown that women are given fewer diagnostic tests than men. This may be because some tests (like exercise stress tests) tend to give more "*false-positive*" results (indicating disease is present when it is not) in women than in men, but it may also be because a healthcare pro-fessional initially dismisses the possibility of heart disease in women. Four times as many men as women undergo coronary by-pass surgery. One reason given is that women typically have a worse outcome and physi-cians don't want to take that chance. But another reason may be that a woman is sicker by the time she is properly diagnosed and treated.

MANY OF OUR HEALTH CONCERNS ARE MISPLACED

We all tend to be victims of the media. It happens easily. The media bombards us with information—information carefully selected by an editor or producer, information that sells—and we jump on the bandwagon. On the subject of women's health, the media bombards us with the issues of cancer and HIV-AIDS. Both, when you think about them, are natural media bonanzas. They offer mystery, suspense, pathos, and drama. Far more than heart disease.

Cancer in particular, has captured our attention. We are riveted on it, consumed by it. In a national survey of women over age 25, sixty-one percent *believed* that cancer was the biggest threat to women's health. But all forms of cancer combined kill about 257,000 women per year—slightly less than half as many as heart disease. Heart disease will kill one in every two American woman. Breast cancer kills 43,800 women yearly, about 1 in every 26 women, and lung cancer another 60,600. Cardiovascular diseases accounted for 44% of all female deaths in 1995. All forms of cancer combined accounted for only 22.5%. And yet we quake in fear about cancer and not about heart disease. We are willing to do almost anything—consume special diets, take numerous supplements, visit holistic physicians, practice unusual regimens of purification—to avoid cancer. Cancer—especially breast cancer—strikes fear deep into our very being, while heart disease doesn't seem to concern us. In the survey mentioned above, only 8% viewed heart and vascular disease as the number one threat to women's health. We pay very little attention to cardiovascular disease. We think of heart disease in women as an oxymoron...it doesn't happen, we don't need to be concerned. And that, of course, is wrong. Dead wrong!

Dr. Martha Hill, a former president of the American Heart Association, believes that the fact that women of all ages and ethnic backgrounds do not fear heart and vascular disease in the same way that they fear cancer "is a major public health problem, because it means that they may not be doing everything they can to prevent cardiovascular disease." Dr. Hill believes there is an urgent need to get the correct message out, and in September of 1997 announced a 3-year national campaign by the American Heart Association to increase awareness of heart disease among women. As the statistics clearly show you, *heart disease is the foremost women's health problem in the United States*. But there is some good news here. Psssst! Pass it on. Heart disease is a disease of lifestyle—and that means that something can be done about it. If we spent nearly half the time, effort and money trying to prevent heart disease as we currently spend trying to avoid cancer we'd be able to make considerable headway against the disease because...heart disease is preventable.

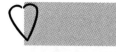

Age-adjusted death rates for women (per 100,000), 1995: cardiovascular disease 135.4 all-cancer 110.4 breast cancer 21.0 lung cancer 27.5

The other media bonanza that is capturing a lot of attention is HIV-AIDS, which, as we all know now, stems from a virus that can be transmitted whenever there is an exchange of contaminated internal body fluids. It is a deadly disease that is altering sexual habits, affecting medical practice, and running rampant around the world. It is currently the eighth leading cause of death in the United States, killing 43,115 people in 1995, mostly young adult men, their sexual partners, the children of HIV mothers, and drug addicts. Most of us feel outrage—for any number of reasons—against this disease, and its astonishingly rapid rise into the Top 10 Killers of Americans.

Compared with heart disease, HIV-AIDS strikes very few women, albeit, young women, and frequently, the babies of infected pregnant women. This is probably part of the reason that the disease receives so much attention. Women (and, of course, children) with HIV-AIDS are typically seen as victims of circumstance.

My intent here is not to pit one disease against another for research or treatment dollars and public sympathy. It is unfortunate that there is never enough of either to attend to all we should. Rather, I am arguing that heart disease in women has never received the attention it deserves—from the media, the medical professions, the scientific literature, or the public. While it is clear that many, many lives could be saved if more attention was given to preventing diseases of the heart and blood vessels in women, much of this energy has been directed elsewhere...often with very little real benefit to the public. We would get "more bang for the buck" with more attention to the prevention of heart disease in women than nearly any other health-awareness or disease-prevention program.

This is because heart disease is different from most other chronic diseases. Heart disease doesn't strike you from the beyond, and you can't catch it—*you earn it.* You earn it with years of physical inactivity, years of poor nutrition, years of stress and tension, and years of smoking. In other words, you earn it with years of poor living habits. You earn it by ignoring the risk factors that most of us know at least a little bit about. You earn it by ignoring basic healthful practices that would add years to your life, and life to your years.

That's the bad news. But there is plenty of "good news" too. You can undo many of the bad habits. You can undo all—or nearly all—the sedentary living, the unhealthful eating, the stress and tension, the years of smoking and other unhealthful habits. In other words, you can change your lifestyle.

This is because the cardiovascular system is the most adaptable system in your body. It responds quickly, and nearly completely. If you are at high risk of heart disease, you can very significantly modify that risk.

Whereas you can do relatively little to assure that you will not get cancer, you can do a great deal to prevent diseases of the heart and blood vessels. And that's exactly what the remainder of this book is all about—how to lower your risk of heart and vascular disease.

CHAPTER 2

Understanding Heart Disease

More than 1 out of 5 American women have some form of heart and vascular disease. This chapter will tell you exactly what heart disease is. It will describe how heart disease develops, many of the signs and symptoms of heart disease and heart attack, and some of the medical conditions that may result from prolonged disease or heart attack. But terminology can be VERY confusing. And, no wonder, this is a complicated subject. The purpose of this chapter is to help you understand the many terms and phrases doctors or nurses use and the medical jargon that you may read about elsewhere or hear on TV.

WHAT IS CORONARY HEART DISEASE?

Heart disease has several names. As defined in Chapter 1, coronary heart disease refers to disease of the arteries of the heart, so it is a vascular disease that affects the heart itself. It may also be called *coronary artery disease*. Another term used frequently is *ischemic heart disease*. This is because disease of the coronary arteries causes a deficiency of blood flow to the muscles that contract the heart (the *myocardium*) and the *cardiac conductive tissues* that are the heart's electrical system, and they are subsequently deprived of oxygen. Oxygen is essential for these tissues to function properly.

All three of these phrases—coronary heart disease, coronary artery disease, and ischemic heart disease—literally mean heart disease.

HOW DOES HEART DISEASE DEVELOP?

Atherosclerosis

Atherosclerosis is a general term for the thickening and "hardening" of the arteries and is sometimes referred to as *arteriosclerosis*. From the Greek words *ather* (meaning gruel or paste) and *sclerosis* (meaning hardness), atherosclerosis is a slow and silently progressive process. It was formerly thought to be the normal process of aging that caused the loss of youthful elasticity of artery walls ("hardening of the arteries"). Unfortunately, considerable evidence indicates that atherosclerosis actually begins in childhood—even infancy—but does not become evident until later life, often during the fourth or fifth decades of life. It is almost universal among middle-aged persons in Western societies, but as you will learn later, it is not inevitable with aging.

Atherosclerosis is the major cause of heart disease. It is a complicated process characterized by the build up of various substances, including fat and *cholesterol* (a fat-like compound in the blood), on the innermost lining of large and medium-sized arteries. Other substances include *macrophages* (cells that clean up bacteria and cellular waste), blood *platelets* (active in clotting), cellular debris (damaged cells or pieces of cells), calcium and *fibrin* (a material required for clotting of blood). The first sign is a yellowish fatty streak on the inside of an artery wall. This soon turns into a raised obstruction that invades the deeper layers of the artery wall causing scarring, calcium deposits, and the accumulation of even more cholesterol and fat. This material, called *plaque*, will partially or totally block the flow of blood through an artery. High blood pressure may develop as blood flow becomes blocked and the vessel walls become rigid. Eventually, bleeding (hemorrhage) may occur inside the walls of the vessel followed by the formation of a blood clot (*thrombus*).

If this process occurs in the coronary arteries, the blood supply to heart tissues is reduced, causing *myocardial ischemia*. Ischemia may lead to a "heart attack" with subsequent damage to heart tissues immediately in the area of the heart served by the obstructed artery. If it occurs in the brain rather than the heart, then "stroke" has occurred, usually resulting in brain damage and some loss of function depending upon the exact area of the brain in which the damage occurs. If it occurs in the kidney, kidney failure may result. If it occurs in the limbs, *peripheral vascular disease* is the result (see below).

Atherosclerosis is a silent, progressive accumulation of fatty substances, cholesterol, and cellular debris called plaque on the inside walls of arteries. It results in reduced blood flow to your heart, brain, kidneys, or lower limbs.

How does atherosclerosis develop?

Atherosclerosis is a complex process that is thought to begin when the innermost, protective lining of an artery called the *intima* becomes damaged in some way. The sort of "damage" we mean here is "microdamage"—possibly a tiny scratch or bump. But, how can the innermost lining of an artery be damaged? The four most likely factors are:

(1) high levels of blood cholesterol or triglyceride (a form of fat found in blood),

(2) prolonged periods of high blood pressure,

(3) persistent exposure to substances in cigarette smoke, and

FIGURE 2.1
Atheroschlerosis

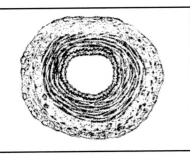

Cross sectional view of normal artery showing the layers of tissue

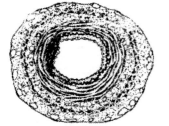

Injury to intima has occured, initiating the formation of fatty deposits and in-flammatory cells on the inner lining

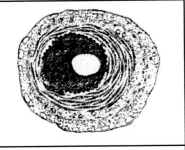

Blood flow is seriously obscured by the formation of plaque

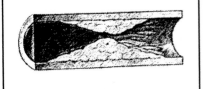

If pieces of plaque break loose, blood clots form and totally block the flow of blood (transverse view)

(4)   prolonged *hyperglycemia* (high levels of blood glucose also called blood sugar) as occurs with diabetes or impaired glucose tolerance.

It is in response to such "injury" that the substances that make up plaque first accumulate on the inner walls of the artery, and some of the fat and cholesterol particles are converted to *oxidized low-density lipoprotein-cholesterol*. This substance—oxidized LDL-C—is an especially harmful substance in the atherosclerotic process.

Note that the culprits that initially injure the intima are the result, in one way or another, of voluntary behavior—of human lifestyle—and hence, are preventable. As Dr. Kenneth Cooper states, "Heart disease is by and large a self-inflicted malady. You don't catch it."

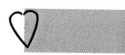

Atherosclerosis can affect large- and medium-sized arteries throughout the body, but a major target is the coronary arteries. Atheroschlerosis is the major process that causes heart disease.

MAJOR FORMS OF HEART DISEASE

Coronary Heart Disease

Coronary heart disease occurs when atherosclerosis develops in the coronary arteries of the heart. One of the most common symptoms is chest pain both at rest and on exertion. This is referred to as *angina pectoris*. Angina is typically described as a squeezing or pressing pain in the middle of the chest that radiates to the neck, shoulders, left arm, or jaw. It happens when heart muscle is deprived of an adequate oxygen supply (myocardial ischemia). Angina may be triggered when the needs of the heart increase, as in physical exertion or emotional excitement, and blood flow to the heart can not increase accordingly. Angina may also occur because of stress-induced spasms of the coronary arteries. All chest pain, however, does not signify heart disease. Fleeting chest pain, or pain with breathing or belly movement, unlike that described above, is less likely to be angina.

The prevalence of angina is higher in women than in men, and is the most common initial manifestation of coronary heart disease other than heart attack. The American Heart Association estimates that 4,300,000 women have angina, but it is a sign of impending myocardial infarction less often than in men. Angina is more likely to predict a heart attack in older women than in younger women. In contrast to men, women who are having a heart attack are more likely to complain of upper abdominal pain, respiratory distress, nausea and fatigue, than the classic anginal symptoms.

Angina is chest pain caused by an insufficient oxygen supply to the heart. It is one of the most common symptoms of heart disease, particularly in women.

Coronary artery spasm is an involuntary contraction of arterial muscle tissue and is thought to be among the causes of angina, sudden cardiac death, and heart attack. It may be caused by atherosclerosis, smoking, and/or stress. This is similar to what happens when a leg muscle does not receive an adequate oxygen supply—and we've all had that happen occasionally. We usually refer to this as a "cramp" or "charley horse."

In severe cases of coronary heart disease, blood vessels may be so narrowed from atherosclerosis that even during periods of rest, the heart does not receive enough oxygen. Sometimes this causes a spasm in a coronary artery, and angina occurs during rest.

A heart attack, or *myocardial infarction* (MI), is characterized by uncomfortable pressure, fullness, or severe angina that lasts more than a few minutes or goes away and comes back. Heart attack victims often clutch their chests, and there are few events more frightening. There may also be a feeling of intense pressure or weight on the chest either instead of the pain, or in addition to it. There may be nausea, dizziness, fainting, sweating, shortness of breath, weakness or exhaustion, and numbness or tingling in the arms and jaw. Some say these latter symptoms are more common in women than men, and that heart attack in women is not so frequently accompanied by severe chest pain. Obviously, heart attack is NOT experienced in exactly the same way by all victims.

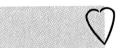

All chest pain is not coronary heart disease, but chest pain, especially if it recurs, should be evaluated by a physician.

Heart attack occurs when the blood supply to part of the myocardium or heart muscle is severely reduced or cut off completely when one of the coronary arteries is blocked—a *coronary thrombosis or coronary occlusion*. The portion of heart muscle that loses its blood supply will die. It is the damage and subsequent death of heart tissue that causes the classic symptoms of heart attack. Disability or death may follow depending upon how much damage results.

In about two-thirds of men with coronary heart disease, heart attack is typically the first sign of disease. Apparently they are victims of *silent ischemia*, myocardial ischemia without pain. So, those who experience angina may be the lucky ones. They have plenty of warning of an impending heart attack.

Data from the Framingham Heart Study shows that about 28% of men and 35% of women had heart attacks that were not initially recognized as heart attacks—they were "silent heart attacks"—their symptoms were not correctly attributed to heart attack either by themselves or their doctors until later. Some women experience a silent heart attack as vague heaviness and fatigue, shortness of breath, and a little lightheadedness, and do nothing about it. Later examination reveals they had an earlier "mild heart attack."

In women, the first sign of heart disease is usually (in about 56% of cases) angina, but as stated earlier, angina does not always progress to heart attack. In older women or women with diabetes, heart attack symptoms may be particularly vague. Vague and unusual feelings in the chest that are persistent may seem pretty harmless, but may actually be a forewarning of a major heart attack. There are probably about a million people in the United States who have no idea (nor do their doctors) that they have significant myocardial ischemia.

Figure 2.2
Heart Attack/Myocardial Infarction

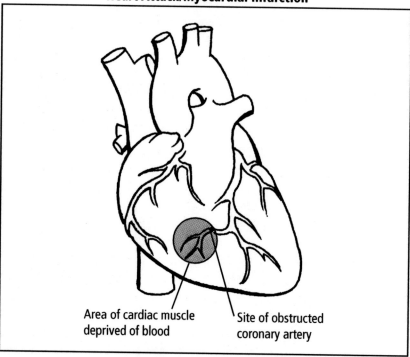

Area of cardiac muscle
deprived of blood

Site of obstructed
coronary artery

The "classic" signs of heart attack:	As a woman, you may have other, less common warning signs:
• uncomfortable pressure, fullness, squeezing or pain in the center of the chest that lasts more than a few minutes, or goes away and comes back. • pain that spreads to the shoulders, neck or arms. • chest discomfort with lightheadedness, fainting, sweating, nausea or shortness of breath.	• atypical chest pain, stomach or abdominal pain. • nausea or dizziness. • shortness of breath and difficulty breathing. • unexplained anxiety, weakness or fatigue. • palpitations, cold sweat or paleness. Not all symptoms will occur in every attack.

Heart Failure

When the heart has weakened to the point that it is unable to pump blood efficiently enough to meet the needs of the body it is said to be in *congestive heart failure*. Heart failure is not a specific disease. It refers to symptoms that occur when the heart is not functioning effectively. Unfortunately, heart failure affects 1 in every 100 people in the United States; 15% will die within 1 year. It obviously, has enormous impact.

The most common causes of heart failure are coronary heart disease, damage from a heart attack, valvular heart disease (page 21), disease of the heart tissue (*cardiomyopathy*) (page 22) and high blood pressure.

When the heart functions inadequately, blood accumulates in the veins (venous congestion) and some of the fluid in the blood seeps through the vessel walls into the tissues, causing edema. Thus, a person in heart failure may have swollen ankles (peripheral edema), fluid in the lungs (pulmonary edema), and other signs of fluid retention (for example, kidney or liver congestion). Symptoms include shortness of breath and extreme fatigue.

Congestive heart failure is usually a progressively worsening condition and is a common cause of death in advanced old age. In younger people, it may occur following a series of heart attacks, cardiomyopathy, damage to the heart valves caused by inflammatory infections (such as rheumatic fever), high blood pressure in the lungs (pulmonary hypertension), or inflammation of the heart valves or heart muscle (endocarditis or myocarditis, p 21). According to the American Heart Association, congestive heart failure in women accounted for 26,800 deaths and 494,000 hospital admissions in 1995. Currently, 2,400,000 women have this condition.

Sudden Cardiac Death

Sudden cardiac death or *cardiac arrest* is the abrupt loss of heart function. The victim loses consciousness and stops breathing. Cardiac arrest may occur in a person who is known to have heart disease, but may also occur in persons who are NOT known to have any form of cardiovascular disease. Sudden cardiac death is an odd term because people do not always die. It is the totally unexpected nature of the event that is key to its definition. Sudden cardiac death is distinct from actual death which is defined as irreversible brain death. Brain death can sometimes be avoided if cardiac arrest is recognized immediately, and the heart started again. In-hospital survival of patients who experience cardiac arrest improved dramatically with the development of coronary care units with bedside monitoring and external defibrillation. Efficient on-the-spot cardiopulmonary resuscitation (commonly called CPR) followed up by highly trained emergency rescue teams with the equipment to apply electric shock to restore the heartbeat (*cardioversion*) has made it clear that the primary issue in cardiac arrest is the ability to reach a victim in time to restore normal heart rhythm.

Sudden cardiac death occurs less often in women than in men, and typically at an age 20 years older than in men. About 40% of deaths from coronary heart disease in women occur suddenly. Nearly two-thirds of sudden death in women in the Framingham Heart Study occurred in those with no previous symptoms of disease—or at least no recognized symptoms.

Most cardiac arrest is due to rapid heart rate (tachycardia) and/or chaotic contractions (fibrillation) of the ventricles (lower chambers) of the heart. The term "heart attack" is not synonymous with cardiac arrest or sudden cardiac death. Heart attack refers to the death of heart tissue due to the loss of blood supply. Heart attack may cause cardiac arrest, but the reverse is not true.

Who is at risk of sudden cardiac death? Underlying atherosclerotic heart disease is nearly always found in victims of sudden cardiac death. A person whose heart is scarred or enlarged from a previous heart attack, from high blood pressure, or from valvular heart disease is at risk. Persons with electrical abnormalities that cause arrhythmias are at risk, such as in Wolff-Parkinson-White syndrome, a congenital condition that causes a short circuit between the upper chambers (atria) and lower chambers (ventricles) of the heart. People without heart disease who use recreational drugs, or experience significant changes in the blood electrolytes (such as potassium or magnesium) from a massive dose of diuretics, are at risk. Occasionally, young women with the eating disorders, anorexia nervosa or bulimia nervosa, have massive alterations in their blood electrolytes and suffer sudden cardiac death.

Peripheral Vascular Disease

Atherosclerosis can cause pain and disability in virtually any part of the body. *Peripheral vascular disease* refers to atherosclerotic conditions affecting the arteries in the periphery of the body—the arms, legs, abdomen, kidneys, etc. (Peripheral means "away from the center" which in medicine means away from the heart, brain and spinal cord.)

Most often peripheral vascular disease refers to an ischemic condition caused by plaque deposits in the arteries of the groin, thigh, calf or feet. If the clogging of these arteries is significant, the result is ischemia in the tissues of the leg that artery supplies. As it does in the heart, this causes pain in the legs—called *intermittent claudication*—brought on by exertion, heavy smoking or exposure to cold. If blockage of arterial blood flow is complete, pain will also occur during rest.

In addition to pain, peripheral vascular disease threatens the health of the tissues served by the affected arteries. The first signs are skin changes (a shiny look or redness) and ulcerations. In severe cases, reduced blood flow in the limbs, particularly the legs, may lead to *gangrene* (tissue death) following even a small wound like a hangnail or blister, that results in the amputation of the dying (*necrotic*) parts. This often occurs in people with advanced diabetes mellitus.

In most cases, clear-cut symptoms—claudication upon exertion— are sufficient for diagnosis of peripheral vascular disease, but if the doctor can't find the pulses in the legs (groin, ankle, top of foot) the diagnosis is confirmed. Even though painful, treatment usually includes walking because it promotes development of collateral circulation (a parallel blood supply) in the affected muscles.

OTHER FORMS OF HEART DISEASE

Not all forms of heart disease are caused by atherogenic processes—those causing the formation of atherosclerosis. You may have heard about many of these, the most common of which are described below.

Disorders of the Heart Valves

Women are more likely than men to have disorders of the heart valves, and especially mitral value prolapse. *Mitral valve prolapse* is a common abnormality in which the valve between the left atrium and left ventricle bulges into the atrium during contraction of the heart. The problem seems to run in families, and in most cases, is perfectly benign. If the valve becomes "leaky" causing blood to flow back into the atrium after contraction of the ventricle, the condition is called *mitral regurgitation.* Symptoms include breathlessness and heaviness in the chest. Most women with mitral valve prolapse do not have mitral regurgitation. If a physician hears a "heart murmur" (a shushing of blood past a heart valve) diagnosis of mitral value prolapse can be confirmed with an *echocardiogram* (see Appendix A, Diagnostic Tests). About 15% of people with mitral valve prolapse experience valve leakage significant enough to consider valve surgery.

Rheumatic fever, fortunately much more rare today than 50 years ago, can cause heart valve damage. Rheumatic fever begins with strep throat (streptococcal infection), which if not treated promptly, may progress into an inflammatory disease that can affect many connective tissues of the body—especially the heart valves. Fortunately, modern antibiotics have sharply reduced mortality from rheumatic heart disease, but when it does occur, it most commonly strikes children 5 to 15 years old. The resulting valvular insufficiency may last a lifetime. The first symptoms are high fever, arthritic pain and joint soreness, shortness of breath, and possibly, chest pain. A damaged valve either does not completely close causing leakage, or will not completely open (*stenosis*) obstructing blood flow through it. Either form of defective valve causes inefficient blood flow from one chamber of the heart to the next, so the heart must pump very hard to move a normal amount of blood through the body. Rheumatic fever most often damages the aortic valve, the valve between the left ventricle and the aortic artery, the massive artery that carries blood to the upper and lower parts of the body. Damaged valves can usually be repaired surgically, or replaced altogether.

Infective endocarditis can also cause valvular damage. It is inflammation of the endocardium (the membrane that lines the chambers of the heart and heart valves) that may occur when bacteria circulate in the blood stream. Microorganisms tend to settle on misshapen or damaged heart valves, so people with congenital defects of the heart valves or valves scarred from rheumatic fever are especially vulnerable. Endocarditis is a major illness that can be fatal. Symptoms include weakness, fatigue, shortness of breath, and sometimes fever.

Cardiomyopathy

Cardiomyopathy is a disease of heart tissue that weakens the heart muscle. Usually the heart enlarges to compensate for its weakened condition. Other adaptations include hypertrophy—a thickening of the cardiac walls. Eventually, these compensatory mechanisms fail, however, and heart failure ensues. Fortunately, cardiomyopathy is rare in women.

Cardiac Arrhythmias

Electrochemical impulses travel over the cardiac conductive tissues and control cardiac contractions. Normally our hearts contract in a top-to-bottom and right-to-left wringing fashion so that blood moves efficiently from the atria to the ventricles and out through the arteries. The vibrations that make up our heart sounds come from the opening and closing of the heart valves as the various chambers contract and relax. This is nicely coordinated by the spread of the electrical impulses. If a problem develops in this complicated system, an *arrhythmia* develops.

There are many kinds of arrhythmias; some are common and benign, and others are serious. Atrial arrhythmias tend to be less serious than ventricular arrhythmias. Often extra beats arise, either singly, or in groups of two or three. These are known as *premature atrial contractions* or *premature ventricular contractions* and are usually benign. However, long strings of these irregular heart beats cause our hearts to be inefficient in pumping blood, and are dangerous.

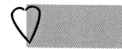

Palpitations are unusual sensations of your heartbeat and are often described as:

- **fluttering in the chest**
- **thumping in the chest**
- **feeling an extra beat**
- **feeling the heartbeat in the neck**

Bradycardia describes a slow but regular heart rate of 60 beats or less per minute. It may occur naturally in healthy athletes, or with heart disease if electrochemical impulses through the heart tissues are blocked in some way.

Tachycardia is the term used for a rapid heart rate (100 beats or more per minute) when a person is at rest (i.e., not exercising). *Supraventricular tachycardia* is a common form of arrhythmia, often affecting people in their 20s or 30s, and causing palpitations, dizziness or fainting. Heart rates may go up to 240 beats per minute. Atrial flutter occurs when abnormal cardiac tissue acts as the initiator of heart rhythm causing the atrium to contract at a faster rate than the ventricle.

Ventricular tachycardia sometimes occurs in heart attack victims, and can recur after recovery too. "V-tach" is a very rapid, regular heartbeat that originates in one of the ventricles. It can be fatal because it so severely reduces the pumping efficiency of the heart. Electrical shock paddles can be used to shock the electrical system of the heart back into proper rhythm (like you've seen on the hospital TV sit-coms).

Fibrillation is an extremely rapid and irregular, in fact, chaotic heart beat of up to 600 beats per minute. Of course, the heart does not function properly when fibrillating because it can not pump blood when it is quivering rather than contracting in a rhythmic fashion. A person who has *ventricular fibrillation* experiences almost instant fainting and death unless the heart can be shocked back into a normal contraction pattern, that is, it is defibrillated. Most sudden cardiac death is thought to be due to ventricular fibrillation. Atrial fibrillation, on the other hand, is not usually fatal, but typically causes fainting, and sometimes stroke. *Atrial fibrillation* often occurs in women over 60, and may be acute or chronic. It often occurs with medical conditions such as high blood pressure, an overactive thyroid gland, or heart disease.

How do you know if a particular arrhythmia is dangerous? Nearly everywoman will experience an arrhythmia at some time in her life, usually in the form of an extra beat. Clearly, not every woman needs treatment. Usually we are not aware of our heartbeat. *Palpitations*, a sensation of an irregular, hard or pounding feeling in the chest, are a common symptom of an arrhythmia. If these are frequent, or particularly disturbing, an arrhythmia may be significant. If there is dizziness or fainting, even without palpitations, then the arrhythmia is most likely of medical significance. A woman should always seek medical evaluation if she has shortness of breath, lightheadedness, fainting, or more than a few seconds of palpitations. If your heart rate is more than 100 beats per minute and you are not exercising, you should seek medical evaluation.

If one of these forms of heart disease is suspected, a number of diagnostic tests may be performed. These are described in Appendix A, Diagnostic Tests.

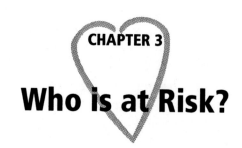

CHAPTER 3

Who is at Risk?

It is becoming more and more clear today that our living habits greatly affect our health, especially during middle-age. To that end, the primary message of this book is that your lifestyle is a major determinant of whether or not you develop cardiovascular disease.

There is compelling evidence that cardiovascular disease is preventable. But to prevent it, you need to know what to do to effect that prevention, and that requires knowledge about the established risk factors for these diseases. In addition, you then need to personalize that knowledge and incorporate it into your life. Chapter 2 focused on describing cardiovascular diseases in women. The purpose of the present chapter is to describe the risk factors for heart disease, to explain how some of these factors are related to one another, and to show you how they particularly apply to women. Chapter 4 will go a step further. It will enable you to evaluate yourself—relative to the risk factors described here. After you read and study these chapters, you will have a good idea about your personal risk for heart disease...for the rest of your life. By the time you complete the book, you will have all the information you need to make appropriate changes in your lifestyle and behavior choices to lower your risk of heart disease. Let's get started.

RISK FACTORS FOR CARDIOVASCULAR DISEASES

The title of this chapter asks the question, "WHO IS AT RISK"—of heart disease? It is obvious that many of us are. I've already pointed out that heart disease is the number one killer of women and that cardiovascular diseases kill more women than all the other major causes of death combined. So, who is at risk? Essentially ALL OF US—EVEN YOU may be at risk.

But how, specifically, is risk for heart disease determined? The answer is that we evaluate your risk factors. So, what is a risk factor? A risk factor is an attribute, a characteristic, or a behavior that research has shown to be highly associated with an increased incidence of disease. Note I said "associated" with increased incidence, the number of new cases of the disease. I want to be very clear about the difference between "associated" variables or factors and "causal" variables or factors. "Cause" is very difficult to determine, especially in chronic diseases (as opposed to infectious diseases) that tend to be linked with increasing age. To be "associated with" means "linked with" or "seen in conjunction with." I am not trying to be obtuse here, it's just that causation is quite a bit different from "associated with," and risk factors are attributes or variables that may or may not be "causal" factors in a disease. Let's see if an example about an infectious disease helps clear up what a risk factor is...and is not.

Medical science has revealed that to catch a common cold a person must come into contact with a cold virus. The virus "causes" the cold. That is now well established. A risk factor for a common cold may be exposure to a large number of people in an enclosed space. Why? Because the cold virus is more likely to be present whenever a large number of people are together and the virus is more likely to be dispersed among them if they are in an enclosed space. "Being with a large number of people in an enclosed space" is not the *cause* of catching a cold, but it greatly *increases your risk* of catching a cold. The point here is that a risk factor may not be a cause of a particular disease, but statistics show that it *greatly increases your odds* or "chances"—your risk—of getting that particular disease.

Numerous risk factors have been identified for heart disease. The American Heart Association has classified these risk factors into "major risk factors" and "contributing risk factors," and also into "non-modifiable," that is you can't change them, and "modifiable," you can change them. At

Major risk factors for heart disease

Non-modifiable risk factors:

- **Increasing age**
- **Being male**
- **Family history (heredity)**

Modifiable risk factors:

- **Cigarette smoking**
- **High blood cholesterol (hyperlipidemia)**
- **High blood pressure (hypertension)**
- **Physical inactivity**

Contributing risk factors:

- **Diabetes**
- **Obesity**
- **Stress response**

(The American Heart Association, 1996)

least two of the "contributing" risk factors may be more important for women than for men. Each well-established risk factor will be discussed here, but the modifiable risk factors will be discussed in greater detail. Obviously, the risk factors that are modifiable are of most interest because you can do something about them, and reduce your risk of heart disease. The more risk factors you have, the higher your risk or chance of developing heart disease.

The Non-modifiable Risk Factors for Heart Disease

There are three non-modifiable risk factors:

Increasing age

Although we often wish we could, we can not alter our age. As we get older, our risk for developing cardiovascular disease increases. As described in Chapter 2, atherosclerosis begins in childhood and progresses gradually, often manifesting itself in middle-age. For women, age-specific risk of

Figure 3.1:
Mortality rates from heart disease for
US males and females as a function of age.

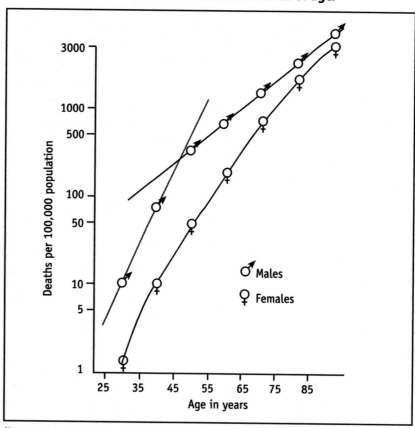

(Barrett-Connor, 1997, p 256. Permission granted by the publisher.)

cardiovascular disease is lower than for men at any age, but after about age 55, the difference is significantly reduced, and thus, being older than 55 is considered a major risk factor for women.

The theory that *endogenous* estrogen (the estrogen the body naturally produces) protects a woman from cardiovascular disease has often been used to explain why women develop heart disease 10 to 20 years *after* men do. And, because age 51 or 52 is about when menopause occurs, menopause has often been used as the explanation for the increased risk of heart disease in women after age 55. However, if the loss of endogenous estrogen was the explanation for the increase in heart disease with age, there would be a sudden increase in heart disease after menopause when endogenous estrogen declines. As you can see from Figure 3.1, that is not the case. There is not a sudden increase in heart disease following menopause. Rather, the risk of heart disease increases continuously throughout the life span. I think menopause has gotten a bum rap. I will discuss the role of estrogen in heart disease more fully in Chapter 5.

Being male

The male death rate (the number of deaths per 100,000 population) from coronary heart disease exceeds the female death rate at every age. This universal advantage of women has never been fully explained. As mentioned above, the obvious explanation is that estrogen is good and that testosterone is bad, but Figure 3.1 does not support this. Other explanations have been offered. For example, that men have inherently less healthy behaviors; that men are more aggressive and competitive and more prone to the consequences of stress; that men have fewer socialization and communication skills, and thus, less social support, which appears to be cardioprotective; and also that more men have high blood pressure and high blood cholesterol. However, none of these differences entirely explain sex differences in mortality from heart disease, and the phenomenon remains largely unexplained.

Family history (heredity)

There seems to be a genetic tendency or predisposition to develop heart or vascular disease. The clustering of heart disease in families has been recognized for some time. Inherited genes apparently make you more susceptible to the atherosclerotic process and in particular, your ability to produce cholesterol and lipoproteins. Familial high cholesterol is well established. Other inherited traits may contribute to the development of high blood pressure, diabetes, obesity, and specific patterns of body fat distribution. Without genetic testing, you don't know if you have inherited these factors, but statistics show that you are at increased risk if one or both of your biological parents had cardiovascular disease at an early age. Usually this means before age 55.

Race or ethnic background is a factor as well. African-Americans have a higher risk of developing high blood pressure than white Americans and this makes them highly susceptible to heart disease. Black women have a death rate from high blood pressure that is almost five times higher than the rate in white women. For heart disease, black women die at 1.3 times the rate of white women. Hispanic women, on the other hand, have about one-third the death rate from heart disease as white women.

But families pass on more than genes. Many behaviors learned in childhood are carried on into adult life. What you eat, your exercise patterns, and your drinking and smoking habits, for example, are strongly influenced by your early family life. These behaviors, either directly or indirectly, affect many of the modifiable risk factors.

Having non-modifiable risk factors does not mean that cardiovascular disease is inevitable or guaranteed. But if you have non-modifiable risk factors—for example, a parent who died of heart disease, and you are over age 55—then it is particularly important for you to lower your modifiable risk factors. These risk factors are strongly affected by your lifestyle and health behaviors. Some of them can be altered by taking medications, but medication always carries a certain risk and I've never yet heard of a drug that didn't have some sort of side effect. But, more on the advantages of lifestyle changes over drug therapies later. Let's turn our attention to the modifiable risk factors for heart disease.

The Modifiable Risk Factors for Heart Disease

The risk factors discussed below can, for the most part, be altered with your lifestyle. This is the primary message of this book—that you can do something about these factors and lower your risk of heart disease. Even if you are at the high risk end of the continuum relative to the non-modifiable risk factors, it is not inevitable that you will get cardiovascular disease. Your behavior has much to do with this. And, even if you score high on a number of the following risk factors today, you can change that.

Smoking

In her book *All About Eve*, Tracy Semler writes "Smoking is suicide for women." (p. 386) And nothing could be closer to the truth. I think about everyone knows that smoking is closely associated with lung cancer, but it is also closely associated with chronic respiratory diseases such as emphysema and asthma, a high risk of pneumonia, increased risk during surgery, headaches and ulcers, and a four-fold risk of Alzheimer's disease. Do I have your attention yet? If you're a smoker, I sure hope so. There is also a strong relationship between smoking (both cigarettes and cigars) and heart disease.

According to the 1997 statement of the American Heart Association on cardiovascular disease in women, smoking is "the leading preventable cause of heart disease in women." More than half of the myocardial infarctions among middle-aged women each year are attributable to tobacco. The excess risk of heart disease due to smoking is between two- and four-fold, and it is even higher for stroke. This makes smoking the most important risk factor for heart disease—it accounts for more excess risk than any other risk factor.

The health risks associated with smoking are usually said to be "dose related"—which means that the more cigarettes smoked daily, the higher the risk. The Nurses' Health Study indicates that even "a little smoking" is dangerous. Results show that just 1 to 4 cigarettes a day *doubles* a woman's risk of heart attack. Smokers also are six times more likely to die when they have a heart attack than are non-smokers—six times more likely!

What is it about smoking that is so highly related to heart disease? Gosh, where do I begin! I'll only cover the effects of smoking that are most directly related to heart disease (otherwise I'd have to write a whole book), and none of those related to the numerous respiratory problems it causes (which, incidently, also affect the heart because respiratory problems usually force the heart to work harder than necessary).

Tobacco smoke contains over 2000 known substances including nicotine, carbon monoxide, nitrogen dioxide, benzine, formaldehyde, and hydrogen cyanide. Nicotine and carbon monoxide are known to damage the innermost lining of arteries. First, nicotine stimulates the smooth muscles in arterial walls causing them to contract. This narrows the vessels resulting in reduced blood flow to the arms and legs and internal organs (the brain, the heart itself, the kidney, etc). Thus the cells of your body receive less blood flow, and consequently, lesser amounts of the nutrients and oxygen that it carries. Smoking is the biggest risk factor for peripheral vascular disease, and in fact, the condition is almost exclusively found in smokers. Smokers with peripheral vascular disease are more likely, too, to develop gangrene and require leg or foot amputation than nonsmokers.

Nicotine usually causes blood pressure to rise and the heart to beat faster, partly the result of the physiological responses just mentioned, and partly because nicotine stimulates the adrenal glands and the release of adrenaline. This is part of the "upper" or stimulating effect of nicotine. Smoking also increases the likelihood of cardiac arrhythmias and coronary artery spasms, which are closely related to increased incidence of sudden cardiac death. The increase in heart rate and blood pressure increases the work the heart has to do, and consequently, its need for oxygen, which is probably no problem for a young, healthy heart...but, if there is illness, or atherosclerosis...

Smoking reduces the oxygen-carrying capacity of blood. This means that a given quantity of blood carries less oxygen in a smoker than in a nonsmoker. This happens because inhaled cigarette (or cigar) smoke contains a large amount of carbon monoxide (yes, the stuff that causes carbon monoxide poisoning). This gas is VERY readily absorbed into your blood where it is taken up by your red blood cells. In smokers, approximately 5 to 10% of the red blood cells are immobilized by carbon monoxide—that means they can't carry the oxygen they are supposed to be carrying to your cells; nor can they remove carbon dioxide.

Smoking is a major cause of the microdamage to the inner surface of your arteries that initiates the development of atherosclerosis. This is probably the primary reason that smoking is the most significant risk factor for heart attack.

Cigarette smoke causes blood platelets to become sticky and cluster together. This increases blood thickness and shortens clotting time. Consequently, the risk of thrombosis increases with smoking, and particularly in women who also use oral contraceptives ("the pill"). Research clearly shows that smoking, combined with oral contraceptives, increases the risk of heart disease many, many times over.

Smoking acts synergistically with other risk factors too, but not in an additive way, in a multiplicative way! Smokers who also have hypertension (our next topic) or high cholesterol, have greatly increased risk of heart disease and stroke.

But who smokes anymore? I'm sorry to report, that although there has been a significant decline in smoking since the 1988 Surgeon General's Report on the health dangers of smoking and the addicting effects of nicotine, there are still 23.5 million women smokers in the United States. That's 25% of white women, 22% of black women, and 15% of Hispanic women. In addition, 4.4 million teenagers between 12 and 17 smoke, and most of these are girls. That's far, far too many! The Centers for Disease Control and Prevention report that 61,000 American women over the age of 35 died from cardiovascular diseases attributable to cigarette smoking in 1990. There is simply no doubt about it (even though the tobacco companies still contest it)—smoking is the single greatest cause of preventable death in the United States! And the low-tar, low-nicotine cigarettes especially marketed for women are just as dangerous.

If you smoke, you MUST stop. And you may need help. Most people do. The Surgeon General warned that nicotine is highly addicting, as addicting as heroin or cocaine, and consequently, one of the most difficult of addictions to break. But this life-threatening addiction CAN be stopped.

Here is some good news. Even in heavy smokers, risk declines rapidly once they've stopped smoking. Three years after quitting, the risk of death from heart disease and stroke—even in people who smoked as much as a-pack-a-day, is almost the same as in people who never smoked at all.

How to quit. There are many ways to quit. Although some people can go "cold turkey" and quit smoking abruptly, most can not. I suggest you find a successful smoking cessation program and join it. A program with good results is Smokers Anonymous.

You may want to try easing down the nicotine levels in your blood by using nicotine chewing gum, or the nicotine patch. You'll have to consult your doctor to get the nicotine patch—its a prescription medication.

Whatever method you try, I highly recommend getting some good advice and reading up on the topic. Go to your local library. (I'm told the book *How Women can Stop Smoking* by Robert Klesges & Margaret DeBon is quite helpful.) Call the closest branch of the American Cancer Society and American Lung Association (see Resources). They not only have smoking cessation programs but smoking cessation literature.

What about weight gain? One of the primary deterrents to smoking cessation is that women often gain weight when they quit smoking. But this varies considerably from woman to woman. Some women gain 10 pounds, other women none at all. Many women claim that they smoke to keep their weight down. This is a prime example of being "pound foolish," of being more concerned about cosmetic appearance than the health impact of smoking. If you smoke to keep your weight down, please review the facts. There is far more danger involved in smoking than there is in carrying a few extra pounds. And there are far, far better ways to lose weight or to control your weight than smoking. The Heart Healthy Habits program described in Part II will help you. Please quit smoking. In the meantime, read on.

Second-hand smoke. Before I leave this topic, I also want to warn you of the dangers of secondhand smoke (some call it environmental smoke or "passive" smoking). The American Heart Association reports that death from coronary heart disease is increased by 30% in those exposed to secondhand smoke at home or at work. Unfortunately, 47.7% of working adults, and 37.4% of all adults who do not use tobacco, report routine exposure to secondhand smoke at work or at home. The Environmental Protection Agency recently classified tobacco smoke as a Class A Carcinogen to which there is no safe level of exposure.

Perhaps all this will stimulate you to some political activism against the tobacco industry. Here are a few bits of information to chew on a little.

- Tobacco companies have specifically targeted women and teenagers. The ads of such brands as Virginia Slims ("You've come a long way baby") and Ultra Lights promise women the coveted qualities of slimness, beauty, sex appeal, success, and personal intrigue. The "Joe Camel" ads recently outlawed emphasized "coolness" and independence to teenaged girls. Who could doubt that appeal?

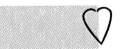

Smoking increases your heart rate and blood pressure causing your heart to work harder and to need more oxygen, but at the same time, smoking decreases the amount of oxygen in your blood.

Smoking initiates atherosclerosis by causing micro-injury to the innermost lining of your arteries.

- The American Cancer Society reports that in women between 35 and 44 who smoke more than two packs a day, cigarette-related medical costs and lost work will add up to an average of $20,152 over a lifetime.

- The CDC estimated that total direct costs for smoking-related medical care was $34 BILLION in 1985.

- The after-tax profits of tobacco companies that manufactured cigarettes in 1989 were $7 BILLION.

- The ads that encourage us to smoke cost tobacco companies $4 BILLION a year.

SMOKING SEEMS LIKE A VERY EXPENSIVE WAY TO DIE.

High Blood Pressure/hypertension

Blood pressure is the result of two forces—one created by the heart as it pumps blood into the arteries, the other created by the resistance of these vessel walls as blood flows through them. The major artery leading from the heart—the aorta—has a vast network of smaller and smaller vessels called *arterioles* which distribute blood within the body. Blood pressure can be compared to the pressure of water coming from a garden hose with a nozzle attached. The arterioles function like the nozzle as they dilate (open up) or constrict (close down). When they are open wide or dilated, pressure against the artery walls is reduced. When they are tightened or constricted, the pressure is increased. High blood pressure (hypertension) occurs when the arterioles remain constricted over a period of time creating a condition that resists the flow of blood from the heart (remember the nozzle on the garden hose). This forces the heart to work extra hard to deliver blood, oxygen, and nutrients to the cells of the body.

Arterioles dilate or constrict on command from the central nervous system in response to all sorts of stimuli. Examples of these stimuli are the time of day (blood pressure is usually highest in the morning), emotional stress (blood pressure rises in a "fight or flight" response), body position (a sudden change from lying to standing alters blood distribution), and exercise (blood pressure increases with exertion). The regulation of blood pressure is complex, but it is known that many biochemical and mechanical mechanisms of the heart, brain, kidneys, and adrenal glands are involved.

When blood pressure is measured, two numbers are obtained. When recorded you see these numbers separated by a slash; for example, 140/90. The unit of measurement is millimeters of mercury (mm Hg), but your doctor probably will tell you the numbers without the unit of measurement. The first, or higher number is the *systolic pressure*, which indicates the maximum pressure of the blood flow when your heart contracts. The second, or lower number is the *diastolic pressure*, which indicates the minimum pressure of the blood flow between heart beats when the heart and vessels are most relaxed. For most adults, a blood pressure reading of 120 over 70 mm Hg indicates a "normal" blood pressure. The American Heart Association defines hypertension as systolic pressure of 140 mm Hg or more and/or diastolic pressure of 90 mm Hg or more for extended periods of time. You are said to have hypertension if either one of these numbers is higher than what is considered "normal" or healthy. About 50 million Americans over age 6 have hypertension—that's one in four! In 1995, 23,321 women died of high blood pressure, and it was a contributing factor in many, many more deaths (stroke, for example). African-Americans are at particularly high risk for hypertension and develop it much earlier in life than whites. This contributes very significantly to their higher rates of heart disease, stroke, and end-stage-renal-disease compared to whites.

I mentioned above that the regulation of blood pressure was extremely complex. The cause of 90 to 95% of hypertension is unknown and is referred to as *essential hypertension*. When hypertension is known to be caused by a specific medical problem such as a tumor of the adrenal gland, or kidney disease, it is called *secondary* hypertension because it is due to or secondary to another disease.

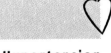

	SYSTOLIC PRESSURE	DIASTOLIC PRESSURE
Normal Blood pressure	< 130	< 85-90
High Normal	130-139	85-89
Hypertension	140	> 90
Stage 1 (mild)	140-159	90-99
Stage 2 (moderate)	160-179	100-109
Stage 3 (severe)	180-209	110-119
Stage 4 (very severe)	210	> 120

(American Heart Association, and National High Blood Pressure Education Program)

Hypertension increases your risk of heart disease 2- to 4-fold and your risk of stroke as much as 7-fold.

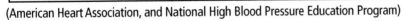

Why is hypertension bad? Hypertension means that the heart is working harder than it should have to. This puts both the heart and the blood vessels under considerable strain. If hypertension is not treated, the inner walls of blood vessels may become scarred, hardened and less elastic. This causes microdamage to the inner surfaces of the arteries and arterioles, and significantly contributes to atherosclerosis. Eventually, hypertension may cause the heart to become enlarged and weakened from having to work so hard.

When elevated blood pressure is sustained over several years, pathological changes occur in the blood vessels and organs, especially the heart, brain, kidneys, and eyes. These changes may be the direct effect of the elevated pressure or the indirect consequences of injury to blood vessel walls. And, unfortunately, there may be no symptoms until the damage is quite extensive—and irreversible. For that reason, hypertension is often referred to as the "silent killer" because there are no outward symptoms. Most people do not realize they have it until a heart attack or stroke occurs. By that time, it may be too late to undo the damage to the heart and blood vessels.

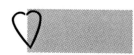

You should have your blood pressure checked at least once a year.

Hypertension increases your risk of coronary heart disease two- to four-fold, and of stroke as much as 7-fold. In non-smokers, hypertension may be the most important risk factor for heart attack. Hypertension is clearly the most important risk factor for stroke—whether you are a smoker or not. A particularly deadly combination of risk factors for heart attack includes hypertension, obesity, smoking and high cholesterol or diabetes. And hypertension also significantly increases risk of kidney disease.

Unfortunately, 60% of white women over the age of 45 are hypertensive. For African-American women, the number is even higher—79% over age 45 are hypertensive. Often hypertension is linked with a predisposition for non-insulin dependent diabetes (sometimes called adult-onset diabetes, Type II diabetes, or NIDDM), high blood cholesterol, and obesity. Loss of weight, alone, will usually do much to correct this.

High blood pressure is 2 to 3 times more common in women using oral contraceptives for 5 years or more than in women who do not use oral contraceptives. Unfortunately, women are particularly susceptible to hypertension during pregnancy, especially during the last three months. If untreated, this can endanger both the mother and the baby. Risk of stroke increases during pregnancy.

For most people, blood pressure increases with age, and in women, the rise is even greater than in men. *Isolated systolic hypertension* (no concurrent elevation in diastolic blood pressure) is fairly common in older women. This carries particularly high risk for stroke.

Hypertension needs to be treated. But recent data indicate that only 66% of people with hypertension are aware they have it, hence the term "silent killer," and only 21% with hypertension have it under adequate control. This is tragic.

The most important thing to understand here is that despite the pathological changes caused by sustained hypertension, successful treatment substantially reduces these increased risks. Lowering diastolic hypertension even by 5 or 6 mm Hg results in a 20 to 25% reduction in coronary heart disease. The same reduction (5-6 mm Hg) in systolic hypertension reduces heart disease deaths by 9%, stroke deaths by 14%, and all-cause deaths by 7%.

Lowering your high blood pressure. There are two approaches to lowering high blood pressure. One is drug therapy—which often involves taking *several* medications, is not always effective, and results in many negative side effects. Unfortunately, most major studies of drug therapy for hypertension show successful reduction in blood pressure, but *no* concurrent reduction in deaths from heart disease. (Drug therapy for hypertension is described in Appendix B along with other Common Treatments for Heart Disease.)

The other approach involves lifestyle modifications that require serious behavior changes. The lifestyle approach to lowering high blood pressure includes reduction of dietary salt, loss of excess body weight, reduction of alcohol consumption, and regular aerobic physical activity. Because the lifestyle approach has no negative side effects, and is quite beneficial relative to other risk factors for heart disease, this approach should always be given an adequate trial before resorting to drug therapy.

The fact that blood pressure increases with age in industrialized societies but NOT in primitive societies, indicates that this increase is not due to age itself, but to our modern lifestyle. An extensive study conducted in 32 countries (the INTERSALT study) showed that lifestyle changes can successfully lower systolic blood pressure by significant amounts.

If you are hypertensive you should seek medical care and alter your lifestyle to include:

- **Daily aerobic physical activity**
- **Calorie reduction if you are overweight (especially lowered saturated fat intake—see chapter 8)**
- **Reduced daily salt (NaCl) intake (if you are salt-sensitive)**
- **Restricted alcohol consumption**
- **Smoking cessation**
- **Relaxation or stress reduction activities**

One of the most effective components in the reduction of hypertension is loss of body weight. Losing weight by simultaneously lowering calorie consumption and increasing physical activity is a key element. Increasing physical activity, especially aerobic activity (described in Chapter 7), reduces high blood pressure even without a corresponding reduction in body weight.

Reducing your salt intake may also be important. However, many people are NOT salt-sensitive and will not respond to salt reduction. I recommend that you and your doctor determine if you are salt-sensitive before going on a prolonged salt-free or low-salt diet because salt-free food doesn't taste as good and there is no sense denying yourself if you are not salt-sensitive.

Reduction of excess alcohol intake is important too. Excess alcohol for women probably means more than one drink per day on a regular basis. Moderate alcohol consumption is of little concern.

Hypertensive people are often high strung and tense, but we can not prove that stress causes high blood pressure. High stress may elevate adrenaline-like substances that result in constriction of blood vessels. You will learn more about stress in Chapter 9.

Some people require a combination of drug therapy and lifestyle change to lower their elevated blood pressure. If you are hypertensive, do not underestimate the importance of getting your blood pressure under control. The Heart Healthy Habits described in Part II will help you do that.

High Blood Cholesterol

Elevated blood cholesterol is a major and modifiable risk factor for heart disease. But not all cholesterol is bad. Your ideal blood lipid profile should be low in total cholesterol and LDL-cholest-erol, but high in HDL-cholesterol.

I don't think there is anyone in America who hasn't heard about cholesterol by now. It is a VERY important factor in the development of coronary heart disease, and one can not discuss the role of food and nutrition in health without getting into a discussion of cholesterol. I know you all have seen the food labels proclaiming products with "no cholesterol" or "low cholesterol." Hardly anything has been said about cholesterol so far in this book, so consider the next few pages "a primer on cholesterol."

Cholesterol is a fat-like substance found only in human and animal tissues (it is NEVER found in vegetable tissues). It is a major component of atherosclerotic plaque. Research clearly shows that the higher your blood cholesterol, the more likely atherosclerosis will develop and blood flow will be blocked in a vessel of the heart (heart attack) or brain (stroke).

Cholesterol is necessary to sustain life because it builds cell membranes. Your liver produces all the cholesterol that is needed, however, and that's why your diet is so important. A diet that is high in animal fats and cholesterol will raise your blood cholesterol much higher than is needed.

Cholesterol is transported in the blood by *lipoproteins.* These "carriers" of cholesterol differ in their proportionate amounts of fat (lipid, hence "lipo") and protein, and are considered subfractions of cholesterol. A high-density lipoprotein (HDL) contains more protein than fat and is referred to as the "good cholesterol" because having a high amount of HDL-cholesterol has been shown to reduce your risk of vascular disease. HDL clears cholesterol out of your blood stream by delivering it to the liver for eventual removal from your body. A low-density lipoprotein (LDL) contains more fat than protein and has been shown to considerably increase your risk of heart and vascular disease. LDL-cholesterol deposits some of its cholesterol in artery walls, and is particularly prone to oxidation. Oxidized LDL-cholesterol is particularly harmful relative to the development of atherosclerosis, and thus, LDL is referred to as the "bad cholesterol."

There are also some particles known as very-low-density lipoproteins or VLDL-cholesterol. These very large particles are composed mostly of triglycerides, and contain little protein. Your VLDL levels are high following a fatty meal. VLDL is typically not measured in your blood sample, but triglyceride levels are.

CHOLESTEROL LEVELS (mg/dL)	DESIRABLE (low risk)	BORDERLINE HIGH-RISK	HIGH RISK
Total Cholesterol	less than 200	200-239	240 or higher
LDL ("bad") cholesterol	less than 130	130-159	160 or higher
HDL ("good") cholesterol	50 or higher	less than 50	less than 35
Triglyceride	less than 200	200-400	more than 400
LDL:HDL	less than 2.5	—	more than 4.5
TC:HDL	less than 3.5	—	more than 5.0

mg/dL=milligrams per deciliter of blood

It is best to have a low level of total cholesterol. But, in 1995, 50.9 million American women had blood cholesterol values exceeding 200 mg/dL, with about 20% of those having values over 240 mg/dL. Contrary to popular belief, women have higher blood cholesterol than men after the age of 55. A total cholesterol of 240 or more *doubles* your risk of heart disease, but the subfractions of cholesterol may be even more important. High levels of LDL-cholesterol (particularly if the LDL particles are small and dense) are the leading factor in the development and progression of atherosclerosis, and therefore directly related to the development of heart disease. HDL-cholesterol is *inversely* related to the development of heart disease. Therefore, a high proportion of your total cholesterol should be in the form of HDL-cholesterol, and a low proportion should be in the form of LDL-cholesterol. This is assessed by calculating the ratios: LDL:HDL or Total cholesterol (TC):HDL. The optimal TC:HDL ratio for low risk of coronary heart disease is less than 3.5 (this means you have less than 3.5 units of total cholesterol for every 1 unit of HDL-C).

In women, low HDL-cholesterol and high triglycerides are particularly powerful predictors of heart disease.

You should have your blood cholesterol checked at least once every 5 years after age 20. HDL-cholesterol should be checked at the same time. If your total cholesterol is 200 mg/dL or more, or your HDL-cholesterol is less than 50 mg/dL, you should have a fasting lipoprotein analysis. This analysis assesses total cholesterol, HDL-cholesterol, and triglycerides and estimates LDL-cholesterol. For best results, you should fast for 12 hours (no food, just water) prior to your test.

Low HDL-cholesterol is a *stronger predictor* of heart disease *in women than in men*. In the Framingham Heart study, women with coronary heart disease had an average HDL level of 53 mg/dL. The Lipid Research Clinics Study showed that an HDL-cholesterol value less than 50 mg/dL was associated with a three- to four-fold increase in death from cardiovascular disease, and that HDL-C was a better predictor of heart disease than total cholesterol, especially in women over 50. And so too, is high triglyceride a better predictor of heart disease in women than in men. In both the Framingham Heart Study and the Lipid Research Clinics study, women with the highest rates of cardiovascular disease had low HDL-cholesterol (<50mg/dL) and high triglyceride levels (>400 mg/dL).

Generally, having high blood lipids is considered a serious risk factor for cardiovascular disease. However, the picture is sometimes complicated. A triglyceride is the most common form of fat in the blood. Often, but not always, a high triglyceride level is accompanied by a high total cholesterol, a high LDL-C level, and a low HDL-C level. When this is case, there is a high risk for atherosclerosis. When other blood lipids are normal, high triglycerides—alone—are a risk factor for coronary disease only in older, post-menopausal women.

But when high blood triglycerides are accompanied by high HDL-C, there may not be added risk for heart disease. Complicated, eh? A good rule of thumb is if your triglyceride level exceeds 300 mg/dl—you need to lower it by dietary changes and exercise.

Cholesterol and insulin resistance. Low HDL-C and high triglycerides occur most often in women who are also _insulin resistant_. This means that cells no longer respond properly to insulin, which normally allows glucose from the blood to move into muscle and fat cells, thus lowering high blood glucose following a meal. Women with insulin resistance usually have a high amount of body fat distributed on their upper body. They also have small, very dense LDL-cholesterol particles which are a particularly potent form of LDL-C relative to atherogenesis. Taken all together, these factors (low HDL, high triglycerides, insulin resistance, upper-body obesity, and small LDL-C particles) are referred to as "the metabolic syndrome," a strong predictor of cardiovascular disease in women. (See Diabetes section below.)

High cholesterol values seems to begin early in life. Over 31% of white girls and 45.7% of black girls less than 19 years of age have cholesterol values over 170 mg/dL, the equivalent of the adult 200 mg/dL. This indicates the importance of beginning preventive measures early in life. Atherosclerosis has been reported in children as young as 8 to 10 years of age. Our American diet of fast foods is strongly implicated here.

Although less studied in women than in men, lowering high blood cholesterol significantly lowers your risk of coronary heart disease, and the effect may be even stronger in women than in men. For each mg/dL increase in HDL there is a 3% decrease in heart disease risk (2% reduction in men). Said another way, this means that a 10% reduction in cholesterol results in a 30% reduction in risk of heart disease. This means it is well worth the effort required to effect this change.

And it does take some effort.

Lowering your blood cholesterol. The best way to lower your blood cholesterol is by making lifestyle changes that include a low fat-low cholesterol diet and regular aerobic exercise. The typical American diet is high in saturated fat and cholesterol, and so, basically, we should lower our consumption of foods known to contain high amounts of these substances—notably dairy products, red meat, prepared (packaged) foods, and all fried foods. By substituting whole grains, cereals, low-fat dairy products, fruits and vegetables, and vegetarian dishes for foods known to contain high amounts of animal fats, and by changing our food preparation methods to eliminate or reduce "hidden fats," we could considerably lower our blood cholesterol values (A Heart Healthy diet will be discussed in Chapter 8).

The latest studies show that combining regular aerobic exercise with a Heart Healthy diet is more effective than making dietary changes alone. Numerous metabolic adaptations occur when a sedentary person becomes a daily exerciser. Among other important changes, your body becomes a

HOMOCYSTEINE—the latest rage in research on heart disease

An avalanche of new research has suggested that an amino acid called homocysteine plays a critical role in destroying our arteries. Conventional thinking has been that high-fat diets trigger an inflammatory process that causes a buildup of LDL-cholesterol in our blood. This results in injury to the innermost lining of our vessels, and atherosclerotic plaque results. But no one has ever demonstrated that LDL-cholesterol is what initially damages our arteries. Recent studies indicate that it is homocysteine, a substance derived from the proteins that we eat (not fat), that causes this initial injury, and makes our blood vessels vulnerable to cholesterol.

If these reports stand up to closer scrutiny, we may routinely undergo blood tests for homocysteine as well as cholesterol screening. Women typically have homocysteine levels of 6 to 10 micromoles per liter of blood. The danger zone is thought to be above 14 micromoles per liter.

Homocysteine abounds in animal protein. Our liver produces homocysteine whenever methionine, an essential amino acid, is broken down. The vitamins B_6, B_{12} and folic acid cause homocysteine to be broken down and excreted, or reconverted to methionine. For this reason, an adequate dietary intake of B_6, B_{12} and folic acid are critically important because they control homocysteine levels. Studies have consistently linked low folic acid intake to high homocysteine levels, and women have frequently been found to be deficient in folic acid intake. About all that is needed is 400 micrograms (mcg) daily, however, so megadoses aren't necessary. Folic acid is found mostly in beans, grains and greens, so eat your spinach and choose whole-grain breads. The white flour used in the making of most American breads is now fortified with folic acid (beginning January 1998). Orange juice is another good source of folic acid.

Smoking and physical inactivity, both known risk factors for heart disease, have been shown to increase homocysteine levels.

better "fat burner" allowing you to utilize more fatty acids for energy production. Coupled with Heart Healthy dietary changes, you are likely to lose excess body fat as well as significantly improve your blood lipid profile.

Cholesterol lowering drugs are also available, but should be resorted to *only* in cases in which cholesterol is extremely high, in women who have been diagnosed with heart disease, or when lifestyle changes fail to lower cholesterol. Recent research published in the *Journal of the American Medical Association* indicates that only about 50% of women *with* heart disease are receiving cholesterol lowering medications. In other words, women patients are being under-treated. I'm sure, however, that as knowledge increases about women and heart disease, this will change.

For more information on cholesterol and the lipoproteins, see Chapter 5 on Estrogen and Cardiovascular Disease and Chapter 8 on Eating for Your Heart.

Physical Inactivity

Coronary heart disease is twice as likely to develop in sedentary people than in active people independent of other risk factors. As many as 250,000 deaths per year—that's about 12% of total deaths in the US—are attributed to lack of regular physical activity. In 1992, the American Heart Association declared sedentary lifestyle to be a major risk factor for cardiovascular disease.

Because *aerobic* exercise plays a significant role in preventing heart and vascular disease, 30 to 60 minutes of continuous exercise that involves the major muscle groups, such as jogging, running, "aerobics," swimming, bicycling, rowing, basketball, racquetball, soccer, or cross-country skiing, has been recommended for years. It is now known that even modest levels of physical activity such as brisk walking, hiking, heavy house work and dancing—if done regularly—can be protective against heart disease, hypertension, stroke, and diabetes.

Physical inactivity is the most prevalent of all cardiovascular disease risk factors. More than one in four Americans over the age of 18 report no leisure-time physical activity at all. It's paradoxical, isn't it? In a society that seemingly values sports and professional athletics so much (consider the popularity of Monday night football and the World Series, and the salaries reportedly paid professional football, baseball, and basketball players), national statistics indicate that only about 10% of us actually exercise enough to achieve and maintain cardiovascular fitness—and that's only about 30 minutes of daily moderate-intensity physical activity.

Most studies suggest that active women have a 50% lower risk of coronary heart disease than sedentary women, and yet few women exercise on a regular basis. The latest data from the CDC indicate that 56% of white women, 68% of black women, and 62% of Hispanic women have sedentary lifestyles. And our sedentary lifestyles begin early in life. Only 37% of American girls and boys of high school age participate in 20 minutes of vigorous activity three or more times per week. We truly are a nation of couch potatoes watching TV.

And, those who do exercise on a regular basis seem to be mostly— the privileged! Women in the upper income brackets and the highest levels of education are most likely to be physically active. Least likely are the poor, the overweight (no surprise!), and the elderly.

Regular aerobic activity is considered by many healthcare professionals to be the key to preventing cardiovascular disease because it beneficially affects nearly all the modifiable risk factors, and promotes a generally healthy lifestyle.

Let's look at a few specifics.

In 1989, it was reported that total cholesterol and triglyceride levels were lowered with regular exercise, with the greatest benefits occurring in women with the highest, that is the most atherogenic, blood lipids. Another study indicated that brisk walking at least three times a week increased HDL-C in premenopausal women. The Healthy Women's Study that is following originally premenopausal women through menopause reported that women with higher physical activity had the least weight gain and the least decline in HDL-C with increasing age. We also know that pre- and postmenopausal athletes have much lower blood lipids than age-matched women who are less active or sedentary.

High blood pressure, too, is lowered with higher levels of physical activity. This occurred in the Healthy Women's Study, the Stanford Community Health Survey, and the Rancho Bernardo study. More physically active women have lower systolic and diastolic blood pressure than less active or sedentary women.

So, regular physical activity helps us prevent the major risk factors, high blood cholesterol and high blood pressure, and also the contributing risk factors discussed below, obesity, diabetes, and reaction to stress. In addition, physical activity directly reduces risk of cardiovascular disease by slowing blood clotting mechanisms, and by strengthening the heart muscle itself. More benefits of physical activity are described in Chapter 7.

What about other healthy lifestyle factors?

Few physically active people smoke, and most are interested in the quality of the food they eat. Few physically active people consume a really poor diet. So by adopting a regularly active lifestyle, you affect many other well documented disease risk factors.

The importance of regular moderate-intensity physical activity was emphasized recently in the Surgeon General's Report, *Physical Activity and Health*, and the federal guidelines adopted in 1993 endorsing 30 minutes of moderate-intensity physical activity "most days of the week." Part II will emphasize increasing your daily physical activity—not only for your improved health, but for the enrichment of your life.

Well, it has taken us many pages to describe the major risk factors for heart disease and stroke as classified by the American Heart Association. And believe me, that was just a very basic primer on the vast amount of information available on these topics. The rest of this section covers what the AHA considers the "contributing risk factors" for heart disease— all modifiable. I don't like to make a distinction between "major" and "contributing" risk factors for women, however, because these risk factors are not only particularly prevalent in women, but also more important relative to cardiovascular disease in women than in men. Diabetes and obesity may be contributing risk factors in men, but they are of major importance and prevalence in women. In my opinion, the first two factors discussed below should be classified as major risk factors for heart disease in women.

Diabetes

About 16 million Americans have diabetes, with 90% having non-insulin-dependent-diabetes mellitus (I'll use the term Type II diabetes). Type II diabetes is the inability to use glucose (blood sugar) properly because muscle and fat cells are insulin resistant, that is, the cells do not respond properly to insulin. In people with insulin resistance, blood glucose levels remain high instead of going back to normal following a meal, and usually insulin levels are elevated. In Type I diabetes, which is less common, there is insulin deficiency because the insulin producing cells of the pancreas are damaged or destroyed. Without injected or oral insulin, people with Type I diabetes can not utilize blood glucose. They typically have high blood glucose levels and low blood insulin levels.

The chronic high blood glucose levels of diabetes (*hyperglycemia*) damages tissues causing kidney disease, blindness, problems in pregnancy and childbirth, poor healing that may lead to amputation of a limb in response to even a minor injury like a hangnail—and a considerable increase in the risk of heart disease. More than 80% of diabetics die of some form of heart or blood vessel disease.

Diabetes is the fourth leading cause of death in black women, and the third leading cause of death in Hispanic and Native American women. It is classified by the American Heart Association as a modifiable contributing risk factor for heart disease.

Most Type II diabetes appears in mid-life, and affects more women than men after age 45. In 1995, 31,130 women died of diabetes, and it is estimated that 4.7 million women currently have diabetes.

Diabetes increases the risk of heart disease 5- to 7-times in women, but only (!) 2- to 3-times in men. Most likely this is because diabetes increases blood pressure, lowers the HDL-C level (the "good" cholesterol), increases the LDL-C level (the "bad" cholesterol), and increases triglyceride levels more in women than in men. Although we don't know why, diabetes apparently increases the stickiness of blood platelets which causes excessive blood clotting, and increases the movement of cholesterol across the innermost tissue linings of coronary arteries. These actions considerably increase the risk of atherosclerosis and heart disease.

The inability to properly regulate blood glucose following a meal is called *impaired glucose tolerance*, which is a sign of insulin resistance, and often precedes the development of full-blown Type II diabetes. About 20% of middle-aged and older Americans have glucose intolerance. This is revealed in a glucose tolerance test in which you are given a glucose drink after an overnight fast. A blood sample is taken every ½ hour for at least two hours by which time, glucose should return to normal levels. To the extent that it does not, you are glucose intolerant. Many women have impaired glucose tolerance without full-blown diabetes.

I bring this up, because this is all very much related to a special complex of factors that seem to disproportionately affect women—upper body obesity, hypertension, high blood cholesterol, high blood triglycerides, and insulin resistance—that is sometimes called "metabolic syndrome" and was mentioned earlier. It is difficult to determine the actual cause of this complicated scenario, but the result seems clear—a substantial increase in the risk of heart and blood vessel disease. In addition, women with metabolic syndrome often are later diagnosed with full-blown Type II diabetes. Obese women are particularly vulnerable to the metabolic syndrome, particularly if they have an upper-body fat distribution, and so are black, Hispanic and Native American women.

"The metabolic syndrome" is a combination of:

- **Low HDL-C**
- **High triglycerides**
- **Insulin resistance (high blood glucose, high blood insulin)**
- **Upper-body obesity**
- **Small, dense LDL particles**

The metabolic syndrome is a very strong predictor of cardiovascular disease and diabetes in women.

Obesity

Even with no other risk factors, people who are too fat—obese—are more likely to develop heart disease. People with excess body fat often have high cholesterol and LDL, low HDL-C, high triglycerides, high blood pressure, diabetes, and increased strain on the heart. Obesity is a risk factor for both heart disease and stroke.

Overweight means weighing more than 120% of your desirable weight for height, or having a Body Mass Index (BMI) greater than 27 (BMI = weight in pounds X 703, divided by height in inches squared). Obesity means you have excess body fat. The two are usually synonymous—that is, if you are overweight you probably have too much body fat (unless you are a muscular athlete).

Figure 3.2:
Patterns of obesity.
Upper and lower body fat distributions.

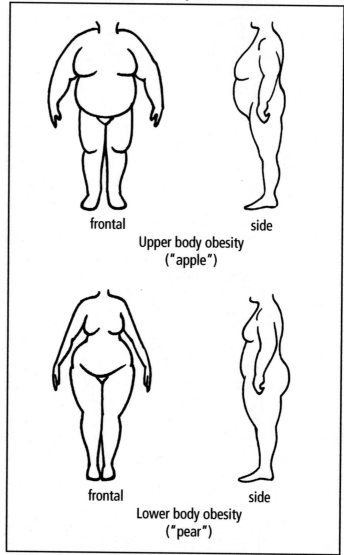

frontal   side
Upper body obesity
("apple")

frontal   side
Lower body obesity
("pear")

(Redrawn from figures in Kavanaugh {1992} and Nieman {1996}.)

Unfortunately, 33.9 million American women are 20% or more over their desirable weight for height. In adult women, 34% of white women are obese, as are 50% of black women, 48% of Mexican-American women, and about 22% of adolescent girls between 12 and 19.

The number of women gaining weight each year is highest in young women. Thirty-seven percent of American women between 25 and 44 gain 5 to 15% of their body weight over a 10-year period. Major weight gain—

over 30 pounds—occurs in 8% of women between 25 and 34 years. And weight gain in adulthood frequently leads to insulin resistance, and eventually, diabetes.

Physicians sometimes seem less concerned about obesity in women than in men because many women carry their fat in their lower body—the thighs and buttocks. In common jargon, this is the typical "pear" shape or lower-body obesity. Upper-body fat, fat distributed on the chest, waist and abdomen, is more typically found in men. This is the so-called "apple" shape, or more scientifically, upper-body obesity. An upper-body fat distribution results in high risk for insulin resistance, diabetes, hypertension, high blood cholesterol and LDL, and consequently, a very high risk of heart disease. This seems to be because upper-body fat has a different metabolic pattern than lower-body fat. Upper-body obesity, sometimes called central adiposity, is closely associated with the metabolic syndrome. Therefore, excess upper-body fat is considered much more dangerous to health than excess lower-body fat.

However, it is not safe for anyone to be obese—even if the excess fat is lower-body fat. In the Nurses' Health Study, women who were 15 to 30% above their desirable weight had an 80% higher risk of heart disease. And, women who had gained 20 or more pounds after age 18, had double the risk of heart disease.

Much of the excess body fat that occurs in black, Hispanic, and Native American women is in the upper body. This may explain why these women have a particularly high risk of heart disease and diabetes.

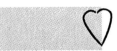

Having excess body fat in your upper body (the "apple" shape) is especially dangerous to your health. It is highly related to elevated blood cholesterol, to high blood pressure, and increased risk of heart disease and diabetes.

Stress Response

Stress response refers to your physical and emotional responses to some external factor. (The American Heart Association calls it *stress reactivity*). The notion that heart and vascular disease is linked to stress has become common knowledge. However, there is no conclusive evidence that this notion is true even though most victims of heart attack state that stress was a factor.

Stress has generally come to mean tension, inability to relax, loneliness, or mental anxiety. Although we all have some concept of stress, it is almost impossible to define or measure it accurately. We all experience stress. Life would be dull without stress. But most believe that too much stress is harmful, and there is considerable evidence to support this.

What stress does to your body. Stress elevates your adrenalin and noradrenalin levels which in turn increase your heart rate and blood pressure. It elevates your blood lipids and blood glucose so they can be used for fuel and increases your blood clotting substances in case of injury. Stress results in the mobilization of your body for action—for "fight or flight." But most often we don't actually fight—at least not physically, nor do we flee. And so these bodily mobilizations aren't used in a healthful way. Instead they contribute to disease processes. Too much stress may cause chronic high blood pressure, speed up the process of atherosclerosis, and increase the tendency for blood to clot. Stress can constrict coronary arteries causing ischemia in heart tissues. Too much stress also leads to unhealthy habits such as the use of cigarettes, alcohol or overeating as coping mechanisms, and sometimes a tendency toward aggressive or hostile behavior. No one doubts the mind-body connection today, and thus few would argue that chronic stress is good for you.

The Type A Personality. For many years, researchers pursued the theory that a hard-driving, tense, time-oriented person was susceptible to cardiovascular disease. The label "Type A personality" became popular lingo for the uptight, excessively competitive, go-getting clock watcher and generally successful social and business climber. Recently, support for this theory has taken a new twist. Originally, the Type A was described as extremely time-driven, always doing more than one thing at a time, for example. Now it appears that the preoccupation with time is not as important as whether the person is annoyed, angry, or hostile toward others. Many time-driven people are successful, happy, well-adjusted and healthy. It seems to be important for people to feel that they are in control of the situation, of their job, or their life. Those who do not feel _in control_ of their lives may suppress anger, or feelings of hostility toward others, may carry a "chip on their shoulder," may feel that no matter how hard they try, nothing will work out right and they will never get ahead. This may be particularly important for women because women's status is often that of the oppressed minority. They frequently work under conditions of chronic discrimination. You've all heard the old adage—women have to work twice as hard to be considered just as good. Or how about: Sweat like a horse, work like a man, act like a lady. Women who work or live under these conditions can't be blamed for developing aggressive, hostile, and angry feelings about their lives. But it sure isn't healthy.

With women's lib, women moved into executive positions in the business world, and many prophesied that heart disease would increase to the same levels as occurs in men. Many believed that women would not be able to hold up to the daily tensions and stresses of decision making and economic tension. It has become quite evident, however, that most women executives thrive on the job. They are quite healthy; they tend to eat well, exercise regularly, and take good care of themselves. The women in the working world who do not do well, it turns out, are women in low-prestige and low-paying positions, who must routinely punch the clock, who have little to say about their jobs and how they are done, and who have little control over their working welfare. They tend to dislike their jobs, and stay in them only because they feel they have no other choice.

There are many ways to break the link between mental stress and heart disease, and preventive strategies have become widely accepted aspects of programs designed to reduce the risk of cardiovascular disease. Methods range from formal relaxation training and cognitive instruction on coping mechanisms, to yoga instruction, group support, and aerobic exercise. I don't think there can be any doubt about the role of emotional stress in the development of cardiovascular disease, but we need more studies that focus on women. Part of the Heart Healthy Habits program you will learn about in Part II will emphasize stress reduction.

SOME CONTROVERSIAL RISK FACTORS SPECIFIC TO WOMEN

We have now covered all the formally accepted risk factors for heart disease, but a few controversial variables are sometimes considered risk factors for women. Until more research is completed, however, the jury is still out as far as I am concerned on most of these factors.

I've already covered the issue of smoking *and* using oral contraceptives. The combination definitely increases your risk of heart attack by a considerable amount. What about birth control pills without smoking? Some research indicates that young women taking birth control pills have a risk of heart attack up to 3 to 4 times that of women not using them. Remember though, the overall risk of heart disease is very low at that age. One study indicated that women who use oral contraceptives for more than 5 years may have a higher risk for heart disease for up to 10 years after they stop taking them. This is because the synthetic estrogens used in oral contraceptives slightly increase blood cholesterol, blood pressure, and blood glucose in some women, and may also increase the tendency for blood to clot. The new oral contraceptives, however, have much lower doses of estrogen than ten years ago and this probably lessens any danger. Research needs to be done with these lower dose birth control pills relative to heart disease, so as I said, the jury is still out.

Premature menopause (before age 45) or surgical menopause (hysterectomy) may also be a risk factor for heart disease. Women who have had surgical menopause have higher rates of heart disease than women their age who have not had surgical menopause, but no one knows why that is. There are too many factors that may play a part to place the blame exclusively on hysterectomy, and I just don't believe it is worth much worry. I'll cover the topic of estrogen (or lack of it), menopause, and heart disease more extensively in Chapter 5, but all I feel confident in saying about premature menopause and hysterectomy is—no ones knows for sure. I believe the evidence that they contribute to a woman's risk for heart disease is weak.

WHEN RISK FACTORS OCCUR TOGETHER

Many wonder "which risk factor or factors is/are most important?" But the real question should be "How many risk factors do I have?"

It turns out that risk factors are not additive—they are multiplicative! Your risk multiples with each additional risk factor. Having two risk factors does not double your risk—it more likely quadruples it! Stated another way, the more risk factors you have, the more dangerous each single risk factor becomes.

In summary, several risk factors tend to be associated with one another. Physically inactive women are frequently obese and have high blood lipids. Obese women are frequently hypertensive, and are highly susceptible to diabetes (insulin resistance). Women who are chronically stressed often smoke and are frequently hypertensive.

Some risk factors are particularly relevant to women. Having low HDL-C, high triglycerides, or being diabetic is more predictive of cardiovascular disease in women than in men. This may be because the endogenous sex hormones (those produced by the body) alter the atherosclerotic effects of these factors.

This has been a long and complicated chapter. Congratulations on making it all the way through. The next chapter will help you evaluate your individual and unique risk for heart disease.

CHAPTER 4

Your Heart Disease Risk Profile

In Chapter 3, I defined a risk factor as a variable that medical research has associated with a significant increase in the likelihood of developing a disease or condition. If you have a risk factor (or factors) for cardiovascular disease, you are in jeopardy of developing atherosclerosis and of having a heart attack. I also pointed out that having more than one risk factor resulted in a multiplying of statistical risks—not merely an adding up of the individual risks.

Every year, people die prematurely from conditions that could be prevented. Evaluating your risk profile for cardiovascular disease—increases your awareness of your chances for heart disease and enables you to direct your attention to what needs to be done to reduce your risk. Risk appraisal may help you avoid becoming a statistic. But there are several things you should understand before we proceed.

First: Calculation of risk is based on statistical data. "Statistical" is the important word here. Statistics are based on large numbers—of people or cases. The result tells us about the likelihood (or probability) of a heart attack occurring in a large number of people given specific circumstances. For example, we can predict that of 100 women over age 55 with blood cholesterol at 310 mg/dL, x number will die of heart disease within one year. Statistics are good at this. But we need to remember that statistics are bad at predicting that a particular 55 year old woman (let's call her Helen) will die of heart disease if her blood cholesterol is 310 mg/dL.

We can say that Helen is at risk, but we can not predict conclusively that she will or will not have a heart attack. Statistics are no good at all for predicting individual results. They were never developed or designed to do that. So, now we have a dilemma—in this chapter you will estimate your risk for heart disease. Whatever the result, you must recognize it as an estimate based on statistical probability in hundreds or thousands of women—some of whom are like you, and some of whom are not like you.

Statistical probability is obviously not absolute. If you end up with a score indicating low risk—I can not promise that you will not have a heart attack tomorrow. Likewise, if you end up with a score indicating high risk—I can not promise that you will have a heart attack tomorrow or 10 years from now. Look again at my example above about predicting that *x* out of 100 women with a blood cholesterol of 310 mg/dL will die of heart disease. Helen's risk of heart disease is based on the number of women like her that died of heart disease. That's essentially what a risk profile does...it tells you how similar or dissimilar you are to people who died of a given condition. You need to understand this or the results may either scare you unnecessarily or cause you to be so carefree that you totally ignore some important information that could significantly improve your health.

Second: As pointed out earlier, nearly all that we know about cardiovascular disease comes from research either done exclusively on men, or that included very few women. Before we can be confident about applying what we've learned from this research to women, it should be tested using studies with large numbers of women subjects. Some of this is currently underway, but it will be years before the results are available. In other instances, the research will probably never be completed. In the meantime, 500,000 women are dying of heart disease each year. We can't wait.

Most of the risk factors for heart disease identified in men are also known risk factors for women. But it is not clear if the relative magnitude of these risk factors is the same in women as in men. Preliminary data suggest it is not. Some known sex differences were pointed out in Chapter 3. For example, we know that diabetes more significantly increases the risk of heart disease in women than in men. We also know that a high blood triglyceride level is a more significant factor for women than for men, but we know relatively little about the magnitude of risk for other factors. This, of course, is unfortunate, but we must proceed with the valuable information that is available.

Third: Although having multiple risk factors considerably increases your risk of heart disease, most risk profiles can not completely account for this. In a few of the categories in this risk profile, an attempt is made to account for multiple risks, but it is difficult to do this accurately, and so, risk profiles will typically underestimate risk when more than one risk factor is present.

Fourth: The questions that make up the risk profile have not been fully tested. They were compiled from several sources that sometimes interpreted the data somewhat differently. In some cases, I provide you with two sets of parallel questions on the premise that each set includes something important that the other does not. The original sources are given in the REFERENCES for this chapter.

Fifth: I recommend that you discuss your results with your healthcare provider. If you are at HIGH RISK, make an appointment with him or her to specifically go over your results and what you should do about them. When you make the appointment, mention that you want extra time to talk about your cardiovascular risk profile or you may not get sufficient attention. If you are at LOW RISK, discuss the results at your next medical check-up. But don't wait too long. Having a LOW RISK profile now, does not mean you will have a LOW RISK profile next year.

Sixth, and MOST IMPORTANT: You can be in control. If you are at HIGH RISK, follow the program presented in Part II of this book, seek additional medical advice, and become well informed about all your options. You CAN do something about this. You can lower your risk. A HIGH RISK profile does not seal your fate, and neither, of course, does a LOW RISK profile.

BEFORE YOU BEGIN

Your personal risk profile for heart disease will help you plan your priorities and decide what factors you need to change in your life. It is not an exact scientific tool. It is more like a "rule of thumb," a guideline. And of course, the profile is not infallible—your final score may be in error either way.

Note that some factors subtract rather than add to your risk. For example, if you have a high total cholesterol you add to your risk, but if you have a high HDL-C you subtract from your risk.

Most of the risks below you can easily assess with readily available information (you can all weigh yourselves). For others, you will need some special information. You will need to know your blood pressure and your blood lipids. Don't guess, and don't use test results from your physical three years ago.

You Need To Know Your Blood Pressure

Almost any trained healthcare professional can take your blood pressure for you. I don't recommend you use the instrument at the local drug store— I just wouldn't trust it. Your HMO, local hospital, insurance company, or employer's medical office will have someone who is qualified and sufficiently equipped to take your blood pressure—usually for free. Another alternative is a health fair—call your local office of the American Heart Association or the American Medical Association for information.

You Need To Obtain A Blood Lipid Profile

Best results are obtained with a 12-hour fast before your blood is drawn. It's most convenient to fast overnight, and have your blood draw first thing in the morning. Fasting means no food for 12 hours, only water. This is done so as to get the most reliable triglyceride results which are highly affected by what (and when) you eat.

Request that your test results include HDL and triglycerides as well as total cholesterol. When you get those you will probably also get LDL. Request also, that you get a copy of your results. If the laboratory does not provide it, your doctor's office can make you a copy.

Health fairs often provide free cholesterol tests—from a finger prick blood sample. Unfortunately, these tests aren't reliable, and only provide cholesterol, not HDL or triglycerides. If that's all you can obtain, it's better than nothing, but you deserve better scrutiny than that. If your insurance won't pay for it, spring for the extra dollars to get a reliable and complete blood lipid test.

YOUR HEART DISEASE RISK PROFILE

Fill in the appropriate information, or check the appropriate space, for each risk factor. You will obtain a score for each risk factor (there will be nine scores). At the end of the risk assessment form, you will be asked to transfer the risk factor scores to a single score sheet and total them for a final risk profile score.

AGE AND SEX

In women, being older than 55 is considered a major risk factor. In younger, premenopausal women, heart disease is usually not prevalent except in women with multiple risk factors such as a smoker who uses oral contraceptives, or a smoker who is also hypertensive.

AGE AND SEX RISK ASSESSMENT FOR HEART DISEASE:
Female, age over 75   (+3) _____
         age 60-74   (+2) _____
         age 50-59   (+1) _____
         age 40-49   (0) _____
         under age 40   (-3) _____

YOUR AGE AND SEX RISK ASSESSMENT SCORE _____

FAMILY HISTORY/ETHNICITY

Your family medical history of any first-degree biological relative (father, mother, sister, brother) is important because risk factors tend to cluster within families. Heart disease at an early age (usually considered age 55) in a biological family member is a major risk factor for women. A positive family history for clinical evidence of cardiovascular disease, for myocardial infarction (especially death of a first-degree relative younger than 65), or for elevated LDL-C may indicate an inherited tendency for high blood lipid levels.

There is also an inherited tendency or predisposition for Type II diabetes (noninsulin-dependent diabetes mellitus) and insulin resistance. The metabolic syndrome described in Chapter 3, is of special significance in women.

Although not listed as a risk factor, medical statistics clearly show that black women are at special risk for hypertension and insulin resistance. This places them at increased risk for heart disease and stroke.

FAMILY HISTORY OF HEART DISEASE

Do you have a parent, brother or sister who has had a heart attack or coronary by-pass surgery?

father or brother before age 55?	(+2)	_____
mother or sister before age 65?	(+2)	_____
yes to either question above, with more than one individual	(+5)	_____
yes to either question above, but after specified age	(0 or +1)	_____
Do you have a family history of hypertension*	(+1)	_____
Do you have a family history of diabetes*	(+2)	_____
Are you of Afro-American descent?	(+1)	_____

YOUR FAMILY HISTORY/ETHNICITY RISK ASSESSMENT SCORE _____

---

*For the death or serious illness of more than one of these family members (for example, a mother *and* a brother), double your score.

SMOKING HISTORY

Cigarette smoking is related to over 400,000 deaths each year in the U.S., and most of these deaths (43%) are due to cardiovascular diseases (cancer accounts for 36%, respiratory diseases for the remaining 20%). Nearly 1 out of 5 deaths result from cigarette smoking. *Smoking has been declared the single most preventable cause of premature death.*

There is a very definite relationship between coronary heart disease and the number of cigarettes smoked per day; heavy smokers have three times the risk as nonsmokers. Data from several studies has shown that at every level of blood cholesterol or blood pressure, smoking doubles or triples the death rate from coronary heart disease. Smoking is also a major risk factor for stroke.

SMOKING

Smoker, 41 or more cigarettes/day)	(+9)	_____
Smoker, 21-40 cigarettes/day	(+4)	_____
Smoker, 1-20 cigarettes/day)	(+2)	_____
Ex-smoker, quit less than 10 years ago	(+1)	_____
Never have smoked, or quit more than 10 years ago	(0)	_____
Smoker, currently using oral contraceptives, under 35	(+2)	_____
Smoker, currently using oral contraceptives, over 35	(+5)	_____

YOUR SMOKING RISK ASSESSMENT SCORE _____

CHOLESTEROL AND BLOOD LIPIDS

There is considerable confusion about how exactly to estimate risk for heart disease relative to blood lipid levels in women. As described in Chapter 3, elevated total cholesterol and LDL-C levels do not seem to be as critical in women as do HDL-C and triglyceride levels. There is also the question of whether or not more leeway should be allowed with increasing age. I have chosen to ignore the age question below, in favor of emphasizing HDL-C relative to total cholesterol, and including triglyceride values (most risk profiles do not include triglycerides values at all because they are designed for men).

You are at risk for high cholesterol and high blood lipids if you consume a diet that is high in fat (especially saturated fat) and high in dietary cholesterol, and if you are obese. Use one of the following three procedures to assess this risk factor.

---

*CHOLESTEROL AND BLOOD LIPIDS   * PREFERRED METHOD**
If you know your total cholesterol, HDL and triglyceride values, use the following method to assess CHOLESTEROL AND BLOOD LIPIDS:
Total cholesterol: (all values below are mg/dL)

more than 280	(+6)	_____
260-279	(+4)	_____
240-259	(+3)	_____
220-239	(+2)	_____
200-219	(+1)	_____
185-199	(0)	_____
below 185	(-½)	_____

HDL ("good") cholesterol:

below 35	(+3)	_____
35-39	(+2)	_____
40-49	(+1)	_____
50-59	(0)	_____
60 and above	(-1)	_____

TC/HDL ratio:

7.0 or above	(+6)	_____
4.6-6.9	(+4)	_____
3.6-4.5	(+2)	_____
3.5 or below	(0)	_____

TRIGLYCERIDES:

Desirable: below 110	(0)	_____
Low risk: 111-199	(+1)	_____
Moderate risk: 200-400	(+2)	_____
High risk: more than 400	(+3)	_____

YOUR CHOLESTEROL AND BLOOD LIPIDS RISK SCORE _____

Note: When triglyceride values exceed 150, the triglyceride content of the small, dense, most atherogenic LDL-C particles so predictive of CHD, is also elevated. This is most likely to happen in women with high triglyceride values plus low HDL-C values who also have upper-body fat distribution, hypertension, and insulin resistance. Women with these characteristics are at high risk of coronary heart disease.

If you know your total cholesterol and HDL values, but not your triglyceride value, use the following procedure:

First Alternative Method:

In 1994, the American Heart Association developed "A Heart Health Appraisal" instrument they called "RISKO." To use this method, find your total cholesterol (TC) value on the left side of the table below, and your HDL-C value along the top of the table. Your RISK ASSESSMENT SCORE for this risk factor is found where the row and column values intersect. (Example: if your TC is 220 mg/dL and your HDL-C is 40 mg/dL, your risk assessment score is +2 points.

TC	HDL							
	25	30	35	40	50	60	70	80
140	2	1	0	0	0	0	0	0
160	3	2	1	0	0	0	0	0
180	4	3	2	1	0	0	0	0
200	4	3	2	2	0	0	0	0
220	5	4	3	2	1	0	0	0
240	5	4	3	3	1	0	0	0
260	5	4	4	3	2	1	0	0
280	5	5	4	4	2	1	0	0
300	6	5	4	4	3	2	1	0
340	6	5	5	4	3	2	1	0
400	6	6	5	5	4	3	2	2

YOUR CHOLESTEROL AND BLOOD LIPIDS
RISK ASSESSMENT SCORE _____

Second Alternative Method:

Either of the two above methods are preferred, but if you do not know your blood lipid levels, use these questions to estimate your risk.

Which of the following best describes your eating pattern?

High fat: Red meat, fast foods or fried foods daily; more than 7 eggs per week; regular consumption of butter, whole milk or cheese   (+6) _____

Moderate fat: Red meat, fast foods or fried foods 4-6 times per week; 4-7 eggs weekly; regular use of margarine, vegetable oils or low-fat daily products   (+3) _____

Low fat: Poultry, fish regularly with little or no red meat, fast foods, fried foods or saturated fats; fewer than 3 eggs per week; minimal margarine and vegetables oils; primarily non-fat dairy products   (0) _____

(Arizona Heart Institute & Foundation)

YOUR CHOLESTEROL AND BLOOD LIPIDS
RISK ASSESSMENT SCORE _____

BLOOD PRESSURE/HYPERTENSION

Fifty percent of all women older than 20 have hypertension, so it is a very important risk factor. Hypertension sustained over several years is accompanied by pathological changes in blood vessels and often in organs such as the heart, kidneys, eyes and brain. Treatment of high blood pressure can substantially reduce a person's risk of heart attack (and stroke), but the risks are not fully reduced for those with blood vessel or organ damage from hypertension.

You are at risk for hypertension if you are obese, have a high alcohol intake, a diet high in sodium and low in potassium, and if you are physically inactive. Black women are at special risk, and especially if they reside in the "stroke belt" (the southeastern US).

The following is from RISKO, the American Heart Association's Heart Health Appraisal instrument developed for women.

SYSTOLIC BLOOD PRESSURE:
Circle the appropriate score below if you are not taking anti-hypertensive medications and your systolic blood pressure is:

(values are mmHG)	SCORE
125 or less	0
between 126 and 136	+2
between 137 and 148	+4
between 149 and 160	+6
between 161 and 171	+8
between 172 and 183	+10
between 184 and 194	+12
between 195 and 206	+14
between 207 and 218	+16

Circle the appropriate score below IF YOU ARE TAKING
ANTI-HYPERTENSIVE MEDICATIONS and your blood pressure is:

117 or less	0
between 118 and 123	+2
between 124 and 129	+4
between 130 and 136	+6
between 137 and 144	+8
between 145 and 154	+10
between 155 and 168	+12
between 169 and 206	+14
between 207 and 218	+16

YOUR SYSTOLIC BLOOD PRESSURE/HYPERTENSION
RISK ASSESSMENT SCORE _____

PHYSICAL INACTIVITY

Not many people seem to realize just how important regular physical activity is to good health. I suppose that is because of the emphasis on drugs to treat hypertension, high blood lipids, diabetes, and obesity, rather than lifestyle changes.

It is estimated that more than 250,000 deaths per year, about 12% of all deaths, can be directly attributed to lack of physical activity. And the greatest benefit of all from regular physical activity is protection against coronary heart disease.

ASSESSMENT OF PHYSICAL ACTIVITY/INACTIVITY:
How often do you usually engage in physical exercise which moderately or strongly increases your breathing and heart rate, and makes you sweat, for at least a total of 30 minutes a day such as brisk walking, cycling, swimming, jogging, manual labor, etc.?

5 or more times per week	(-1)	_____
3 or 4 times per week	(0)	_____
2 times per week	(+1)	_____
1 time per week	(+2)	_____
0 times per week	(+4)	_____

(from Nieman, D. Fitness and Sports Medicine, 1996 p. 360)

YOUR PHYSICAL ACTIVITY/INACTIVITY
RISK ASSESSMENT SCORE _____

DIABETES AND GLUCOSE INTOLERANCE

Diabetes is considered a *more significant* risk factor for heart disease in women than in men. The factors discussed in Chapter 3—obesity, having an upper-body fat distribution even without obesity, abnormal glucose tolerance, and physical inactivity—not only place you at risk for Type II diabetes, but also exert a strong atherogenic (atherosclerosis-causing) effect. If you have a family history of diabetes, you are at increased risk. The interaction of diabetes and hypertension is a particularly potent combination that considerably increases your probability of developing heart disease or stroke.

If you are overweight, have an upper-body fat distribution pattern, and are over age 45, I recommend that you have a fasting blood glucose test. If the results are normal, the test should be repeated every three years. If you are at risk for diabetes, you should begin yearly testing before age 45.

DIABETES RISK ASSESSMENT

Have you been diagnosed with diabetes by a doctor?

Yes   (+4)   _____

No   (0)   _____

If you answered "yes," skip to the next section. (ASSESSMENT OF BODY WEIGHT/OBESITY)

If you answered "no,", answer the next question:

Do you have impaired glucose tolerance? (a positive oral glucose tolerance test)

Yes   (+1)   _____

No   (0)   _____

If you answered "yes" to either question above, skip to the next section (ASSESSMENT OF BODY WEIGHT/OBESITY).

If you answered "no" to the two questions above (or have never been tested), continue with the following questions. These indicate your disposition for insulin resistance and diabetes mellitus.

Have you had more than one baby weighing over 9 lbs at birth?

Yes   (+½)   _____

No   (0)   _____

Do you have a parent with diabetes?

Yes   (+½)   _____

No   (0)   _____

Do you have a brother or sister with diabetes?

Yes   (+1)   _____

No   (0)   _____

Have you experienced one or more of the following symptoms on a regular basis?

excessive thirst   (+½)   _____

frequent urination   (+½)   _____

increased appetite accompanied by unexplained weight loss

                                       (+½)   _____

YOUR DIABETES RISK ASSESSMENT SCORE _____

BODY WEIGHT, OBESITY AND BODY FAT DISTRIBUTION

Obesity is a significant risk factor for hypertension, high blood lipids and cholesterol, and diabetes. In fact, I have always been surprised that it is not considered a major risk factor for heart disease and stroke (rather than a contributing risk factor), but I suppose that is because it is not independently associated with either condition. As I will emphasize later in this book, you can be fit and fat.

The distribution of your body fat, as explained in Chapter 3, is very important. Having your body fat distributed primarily in your upper body and trunk is far more dangerous than having most of your body fat in your lower body (hips, buttocks, and thighs).

There are two assessment procedures below, one to assess your body weight, and the other to assess your body fat distribution. Complete both. The table below places you in a weight category relative to your height. It "allows" you to be up to 120% of your ideal weight (category A) before giving you "risk" points for heart disease and stroke. The second procedure describes your body fat distribution. I think you will find this quite interesting.

ASSESSMENT OF YOUR BODY WEIGHT
Locate your weight category in the table below. If you are...

Weight category A	(0)	_____
Weight category B	(+1)	_____
Weight category C	(+2)	_____
Weight category D	(+9)	_____

WEIGHT CATEGORY

FT	IN	A	B	C	D
4	8	up to 139	140-161	162-184	185+
4	9	up to 140	141-162	163-185	186+
4	10	up to 141	142-163	164-187	188+
4	11	up to 143	144-166	167-190	191+
5	0	up to 145	146-168	169-193	194+
5	1	up to 147	148-171	172-196	197+
5	2	up to 149	150-173	174-198	199+
5	3	up to 152	153-176	177-201	202+
5	4	up to 154	155-178	179-204	205+
5	5	up to 157	158-182	183-209	210+
5	6	up to 160	161-186	187-213	214+
5	7	up to 165	166-191	192-219	220+
5	8	up to 169	170-196	197-225	226+
5	9	up to 173	174-201	202-231	232+
5	10	up to 178	179-206	207-238	239+
5	11	up to 182	183-212	213-242	243+
6	0	up to 187	188-217	218-248	249+
6	1	up to 191	192-222	223-254	255+

(from RISKO, American Heart Association, 1994)

ASSESSMENT OF YOUR BODY FAT DISTRIBUTION

If you are obese (weight category B and above), you are at even greater risk if your body fat is distributed in your upper body—neck, chest, trunk and abdominal area. Waist-hip-ratio (WHR) is one way to assess your body fat distribution.

Calculating Your Waist-Hip-Ratio (WHR)

Step 1: Using a nonelastic tape, measure the circumference of your waist either at its narrowest point or at the level of your umbilicus (belly button). The tape should be pressed tightly around your body, but it should not depress the skin. Be sure the tape is not twisted. Measure to the nearest millimeter or sixteenth of an inch. Record your measurement here _____

Step 2: Now measure your hip circumference at the maximal circumference of your buttocks (don't cheat now). You will need to stand sideways to a mirror to see where the correct place is. Again, the tape should be pressed tightly against your skin or underclothes, but it should not depress your skin. (Do not measure around anything but your underpants.) Record your measurement here _____

Step 3: Divide your waist circumference by your hip circumference:

Waist circumference = _____ = _____
hip circumference

WAIST-HIP RATIO CLASSIFICATION

low risk	less than 0.80	(0)	_____
moderate risk	0.81-0.85	(+1)	_____
high risk	more than 0.85	(+2)	_____

(from VanItallie, T.B. Topography of body fat. In Anthropometric standardization reference manual (pp 143-149) eds.: T.G. Lohman, et al., Champaign, IL: Human Kinetics, 1988)

Add your assessment of body weight score and your assessment of body fat distribution score.

*YOUR ASSESSMENT OF BODY WEIGHT AND BODY FAT
DISTRIBUTION SCORE* _____

REACTION TO STRESS

There are two general types of stress. One is acute stress. This is sudden and temporary stress such as that caused by an emergency, being caught in traffic on the way to an appointment, or having to make a report to your boss. The significant thing here is that when the situation resolves, so does the stress. Sometimes stress accumulates over time such as that induced by serious financial problems, being caught in a bad marriage, or watching a parent slowly deteriorate and die. This is chronic stress—and far more serious. This type of stress is present most of the time such as job-related stress (not getting along with the boss, the need to sell enough products to make sufficient income, etc.), or an unhappy family life. How people cope with stress varies with personality. As you have seen in Chapter 3, the Type A personality (the time-stressed and goal-oriented person) who is also angry or hostile, tends to develop heart disease. The first 10 questions below are designed to determine if you are a time-driven Type A Personality. They are modified from the original Type A Personality scale developed by Meyer Friedman and Ray Rosenman. The second series of questions, are a thinly veiled questionnaire to determine your "hostility/cynicism" level.

ARE YOU A TYPE A?
check if the statement describes you

1. I always move, walk and eat rapidly. _____
2. I feel an impatience with the rate at which most events take place. _____
3. I hurry the speech of others by saying "Uh huh" or "yes, yes," or by finishing their sentences for them. _____
4. I become enraged when a car ahead of me runs at a speed I consider too slow. _____
5. I find it anguishing to wait in line. _____
6. I find it intolerable to watch others perform tasks I know I can do faster/better. _____
7. I frequently strive to think about or do two or more things simultaneously. _____
8. I always feel vaguely guilty when I relax or do nothing for several hours to several days. _____
9. I am always rushed. _____
10. I believe that whatever success I enjoy is due in good part to my ability to get things done faster/better than others. _____

(adapted from M. Friedman & R. Rosenman, Type A Behavior and Your Health, Greenwich, CONN: Fawcett, 1994)

If you checked 6 or more of these statements you are probably a time-driven, Type A personality.

I am a time-driven, Type A personality.

Yes	(+1)	_____
No	(0)	_____

ARE YOU HOSTILE OR CYNICAL?

1. I have often had to take orders from someone who did not know as much as I did. _____
2. I think a great many people create a lot of their bad luck in order to gain the sympathy and help of others. _____
3. It takes a lot of argument to convince most people of the truth. _____
4. Most people are honest, mainly through fear of being caught. _____
5. Most people will use somewhat unfair means to gain profit or an advantage rather than lose it. _____
6. It is safer to trust nobody. _____
7. No one cares much what happens to you. _____
8. Most people make friends because friends are likely to be useful to them. _____
9. Most people inwardly do not like putting themselves out to help other people. _____
10. People often demand more respect for their own rights than they are willing to allow for those of other. _____
11. I think most people would lie to get ahead. _____

Count your check marks.

Low hostility	score of 2 or less	(0) _____
Moderate hostility	3 to 6	(+1) _____
High Hostility	7 or more	(+2) _____

(adapted from materials from The Preventive and Rehabilitative Cardiac Center at Cedars-Sinai Medical Center, Los Angles, CA)

YOUR TOTAL STRESS REACTIVITY RISK _____

TOTALING YOUR SCORES

Congratulations!! You have completed your personal assessment of the risk factors for heart disease. Now it's time to tally your scores and determine your risk of developing heart disease within the next ten years.

Transfer your scores for each risk factor to the list below so that your grand total can be obtained.

```
RISK SCORE FOR AGE AND SEX                          _____
RISK SCORE FOR FAMILY HISTORY/ETHNICITY             _____
RISK SCORE FOR SMOKING HISTORY                      _____
RISK SCORE FOR CHOLESTEROL AND BLOOD LIPIDS         _____
RISK SCORE FOR HYPERTENSION/BLOOD PRESSURE          _____
RISK SCORE FOR PHYSICAL INACTIVITY                  _____
RISK SCORE FOR DIABETES AND GLUCOSE INTOLERANCE     _____
RISK SCORE FOR BODY WEIGHT, OBESITY AND
    FAT DISTRIBUTION                                _____
RISK SCORE FOR STRESS REACTIVITY                    _____

            YOUR GRAND TOTAL:                       _____
```

LOW RISK: -5 to +5

You are at low risk of developing heart disease within the next five years unless, of course, there are negative changes in your risk factor profile.

MODERATE RISK: +6 to +14

You are at moderate risk of developing heart disease within the next five years unless some risk factors are decreased.

HIGH RISK: more than +14

You are at high risk of developing heart disease within the next five years unless some risk factors are changed.

WHAT YOUR GRAND TOTAL MEANS

It is difficult to be exact about what your Grand Total means relative to "risk category"—that is, where "low risk" ends and "moderate risk" begins, or at what score "high risk" begins. After all, there really isn't much difference between a person with a risk score of 14 (moderate risk) and a person with a risk score of 15 (high risk). Obviously the more points you have the higher your risk for heart attack (and stroke). Any tally of points is too arbitrary to tell the whole story. And so consider the risk categories below a mere guideline, not an exact distinction. If you are in the moderate risk range (a middle range score) for two or more risk factors, you will most likely be in the high risk category. If you have two or more risk factors and by some fluke of scoring you are not in the high risk category, you should nevertheless consider yourself at high risk. Remember I pointed out earlier that having two or more risk factors *multiplied* your risk rather than *added* to your risk. If you are at high risk on one risk factor, but low risk on all others, you will probably find your Grand Total will fall in the moderate risk category.

At the very least I recommend you give very careful thought to your risk placement on each factor. You can't do anything about your age or family history, but you can do a great deal about your smoking, and physical inactivity. You can also alter your blood pressure, blood lipids, insulin resistance, body weight, and level of stress. The purpose of Part II of this book is to provide a means by which you can alter these risks factors (this book will not address smoking cessation—there are other good materials about that). The best use of the results of your risk profile is to identify your status on the risk factors you can do something about—and then act to do something about that.

Remember, you can be in control—if you choose to be—of many of these risk factors.

CHAPTER 5

Estrogen and Heart Disease: What's the Connection?

Estrogen is good for women. It protects them from heart disease and stroke. In this chapter, we will examine the role of the endogenous and exogenous sex hormones as they relate to heart disease in women.

The *endogenous hormones* are those produced naturally by your body. All steroid hormones, a classification of hormone based on chemical structure, come from cholesterol. If we could not make cholesterol, we could not make steroid hormones. The so-called sex hormones—estrogen, progesterone, testosterone—are steroid hormones made by your body, and therefore, the natural levels of hormones in your body are referred to as endogenous. The first part of this chapter will describe the role of the endogenous sex hormones in your body as they are related to heart disease.

Exogenous hormones come from outside the body—you take them as medications. The second part of this chapter will describe the cardiovascular effects of exogenous hormones in the form of oral contraceptives and postmenopausal estrogen or hormone therapy. This section will help you decide whether you should use estrogen therapy during menopause.

ENDOGENOUS ESTROGEN AND THE MENSTRUAL CYCLE

The menstrual cycle has two phases. The *follicular phase* occurs from the first day of menstrual bleeding until ovulation at about day 14 of a 28-day menstrual cycle. The *luteal phase* occurs after ovulation and continues until menstrual bleeding begins again. The hormone profile of the menstrual cycle is complicated and a complete explanation is beyond the scope of this book. However, the brief description below, together with Figure 5-1, will enable you to understand the effects of the endogenous hormones of the menstrual cycle on your blood lipids.

FIGURE 5.1
Cyclic estrogen and progesterone during the menstrual cycle (follicular and luteal phases)

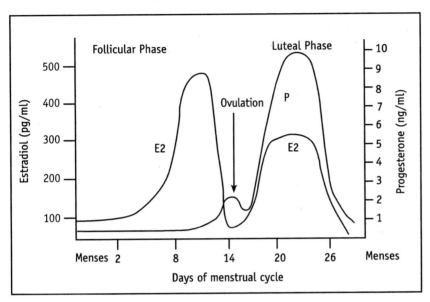

During the follicular phase, your estrogen level gradually increases, but there is little progesterone. At approximately day 14 of a normal 28 day menstrual cycle, ovulation occurs. This is followed by the luteal phase. During the luteal phase, both estrogen and progesterone levels are high. Just before menstrual bleeding begins, both estrogen and progesterone plummet. This triggers a collapse of the enriched lining of the uterus that was built up to support the growth of a fetus. This enriched lining is discarded as menstrual flow, called *menses*. With this as a brief background, we can discuss the changes that occur in your blood lipids caused by these fluctuating or cyclic levels of estrogen and progesterone. Men, of course, do not experience these events.

Estradiol is the predominant form of estrogen in premenopausal women. In adolescence, there is a direct relationship between estradiol and HDL-C. That means that when estradiol is high, HDL-C is high. Remember that HDL-C is the "good cholesterol" because it delivers LDL-C (the "bad cholesterol" with high levels of triglycerides) to the liver for destruction and removal from the body. HDL-C protects us from atherosclerosis. As we mature beyond puberty, estrogen and progesterone establish the cyclic pattern described in Figure 5.1, and although our base levels of total cholesterol and LDL-C gradually increase, they also display a cyclic pattern.

Whenever our estrogen levels are high, the primary form of triglyceride in our blood almost immediately following a meal appears in the form of HDL-C as opposed to LDL-C. After puberty, we see the gender differences in HDL-C and LDL-C mentioned earlier. Women typically have higher HDL-C and lower LDL-C than men because estradiol stimulates an enzyme that enhances the absorption of LDL-C by the liver.

Study of the cyclic patterns of menstrual hormones and blood lipids is complicated and difficult. However, several distinct patterns have emerged. The clearest finding is that total cholesterol and LDL-C is lowest during the luteal phase (by 6-11%). This is because your body uses more cholesterol to synthesize the large amounts of estrogen and progesterone that occur then. Total cholesterol is highest during ovulation, when estrogen falls and progesterone production has not yet begun. (see Figure 5.1) Intermediate levels of total cholesterol occur during the follicular phase. There is about an 8 to 10% difference in total cholesterol between the luteal and follicular phases.

Although less studied, triglycerides also seem to fluctuate with the hormones of the menstrual cycle. Triglyceride levels are highest at ovulation and lowest during the luteal phase.

Women with otherwise normal blood lipid levels have higher blood lipids during pregnancy. All lipids and lipoproteins increase—total cholesterol (as much as 25%), LDL-C and HDL-C (1.5 fold), and triglycerides (2.5 fold). This is considered a normal response to hormone production in the placenta. After pregnancy, most lipid values return to normal, but triglyceride levels take longer to do so, usually about 6 weeks. Several studies have shown a higher risk for cardiovascular diseases in women who have had multiple pregnancies. Whether this is related to the elevated blood lipids that occur during each pregnancy is not known.

During the perimenopause, which usually corresponds to ages 40 through 50, your ovaries gradually produce less estradiol. Much of your estrogen during these years is not produced by your ovaries, but by your adrenal glands and by conversion of adrenal androgens (male hormones) to estrogen by your major body fat depots. This estrogen is in the form of *estrone*, a less biologically active form of estrogen than estradiol. You may miss some menstrual periods during these years, possibly becoming quite irregular. As these events occur, there is usually a very gradual increase in your total cholesterol and LDL-C levels. One study reported a 19% increase in total cholesterol over an 8-year period. At the same time, there is usually a decrease in HDL-C as your endogenous estrogen levels decline.

Menopause, which is the natural cessation of your menstrual periods, typically occurs between ages 50 and 52. Following menopause, estrone becomes the prevalent form of estrogen, and in most women total choles-

With sexual maturity we first see the gender-specific differences in HDL-C and LDL-C. Women have higher HDL-C than men.

As our endogenous hormones fluctuate with our menstrual cycle, so too do our blood lipids. When estradiol is high so are our HDL-C levels. When both estrogen and progesterone are elevated, we have the lowest total cholesterol and LDL-C.

terol and LDL-C increase, and HDL-C levels decline even more. The development of atherosclerosis increases in a corresponding manner. These changes are associated with an increased risk of heart disease of about 25% independent of other risk factors.

I don't want to leave an incorrect impression here. I am not contradicting my earlier statements (in Chapter 3) doubting that menopause was the *cause* of the increased risk of heart disease with age. I am simply stating that sometime after age 40 our estrogen production and HDL-C level decreases, our total cholesterol and LDL-C levels increase, and our risk of heart disease rises accordingly. Our increased risk of heart disease is much more closely associated with age, than with menopause itself.

Estrogen has several other important beneficial effects. Let's examine those now.

OTHER BENEFICIAL EFFECTS OF ENDOGENOUS ESTROGEN

Estrogen dilates blood vessels by causing the smooth muscle cells in the walls of arteries to relax. The result is increased blood flow through the arteries of the heart. During the years when a woman's estradiol levels are high, this is a distinct benefit relative to the prevention of atherosclerosis and ischemic heart disease. Most likely this is why young women have less hypertension than young men.

Also related to the prevention of atherosclerosis is the tendency for blood to clot. Estradiol lowers the tendency for blood to clot by reducing the "stickiness" of blood platelets, and maintaining a major blood clot inhibitor (plasminogen activator). This helps prevent blood clots from forming that are characteristic of atherosclerosis and of some strokes.

Lastly, it appears that estradiol is related to our body fat distribution. Most women, but certainly not all, tend to carry their excess body fat on their buttocks and thighs. The so-called "pear" shape is thought to be associated with the conservation of energy for pregnancy and lactation. Whether it is or not, as many women know, about the only way to lose excess weight from the hips and thighs is to nurse a baby.

The advantage (many women wouldn't call it that) of the pear shape over the apple shape is that fat in the lower body is much less likely to cause atherosclerosis than fat in the upper body, and especially the visceral or deep abdominal fat deposits so characteristic of middle-aged men. During the postmenopausal years, body fat distribution gradually shifts from the thigh and buttocks to the abdomen, and waist circumference increases. The decline in estrogen causes a change in your testosterone to estrogen ratio (your already low testosterone levels do not actually change), and this is usually blamed for the shift in body fat distribution. But the issue needs more study.

HYSTERECTOMY AND PREMATURE MENOPAUSE

Surgically induced menopause occurs when a hysterectomy (removal of the uterus) is performed. When both ovaries are also removed (double oophorectomy), there is an especially abrupt loss of estrogen. Unfortunately for our understanding of this issue, double oophorectomy not only causes estrogen deficiency, but testosterone production also decreases abruptly. Although several autopsy studies have shown an increase in atherosclerosis in young women who had double oophorectomy, other factors were not ruled out, so it is not known whether the reason for the increased atherosclerosis was directly related to the surgery or not. However, population-based studies show increased risk of heart disease in women who have had a hysterectomy. So even though the reasons are not clear, risk of heart disease is known to increase with either hysterectomy alone or with double oophorectomy.

EFFECTS OF EXOGENOUS ESTROGEN (AND PROGESTIN)

Ironically, we seem to know more (but still not enough) about the effects of exogenous hormones on heart disease than we know about our endogenous hormones. These effects depend on the formulation of the hormone, the dose used, the mode of administration, and the age of the user. The information below is divided into two parts because there is a difference between the exogenous hormones taken for contraceptive purposes and those taken for menopausal therapy. Both have interesting—and controversial—effects on our risk for heart and vascular diseases.

Oral Contraceptives

The purpose of "the pill" is to not get pregnant while remaining sexually active. To accomplish this, oral contraceptives suppress the ovaries by providing large doses of synthetic (made in the laboratory) estrogen and its "antagonist," a synthetic progesterone called progestin. A high level of estrogen, even though an "artificial" estrogen, signals the brain to deactivate the ovaries. When on the pill, your body "sees" that there is plenty of estrogen present, and "turns off" the ovaries so they won't produce more. This prevents development of an ovum (egg), so ovulation does not occur. You can not get pregnant.

Oral contraceptives (OCs) were first introduced in the 1960s and at that time typically contained 150 micrograms of artificial estradiol and an almost equal dose of progestin. Almost immediately case reports began to appear suggesting an association between "the pill" and myocardial infarction and stroke. By the 1970s, the estradiol dose had been reduced to

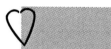

As our body produces less estradiol with the perimenopause:

- our total cholesterol and LDL-C levels increase
- our HDL-C level declines
- our triglyceride level increases
- our tendency for blood to clot increases, and
- we tend to carry more body fat in our abdominal region.

These factors increase our risk of heart and vascular disease.

about 70 micrograms, and a different formulation of progestin was used. Today, some oral contraceptives contain less than 20 micrograms of artificial estradiol, and still newer formulations of progestin.

Only the recent data about risk of cardiovascular disease and the current low-dose OCs is presented here. Much of what you may have previously heard or read is now obsolete (this includes anything before about 1989) because that information dealt with the earlier formulations of oral contraceptive pills that are no longer available. The question here is: Are the current low-dose formulations of oral contraceptives safe in terms of heart disease and stroke?

To answer this question, I will address three issues:
1) the effects of OCs on cholesterol and blood lipids,
2) their effects on blood coagulation and clotting, and
3) their effects on other cardiovascular factors.

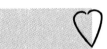

Oral contraceptives, cholesterol and blood lipids

Studies show that oral contraceptives generally increase total cholesterol and triglycerides, but that specific changes depend on the type of hormone formulation used. Estrogen-dominant formulations decrease LDL-C and increase HDL-C, but progestin-dominant formulations either decrease or have no effect on HDL-C. When OCs are discontinued, the altered lipid levels begin declining almost immediately, reaching pre-OC levels in about four to six weeks.

The link between these elevations in blood cholesterol and atherosclerosis seems to be weak. The most remarkable study on this topic was conducted in nine countries of Africa, Asia, Europe and Latin America by the World Health Organization (WHO). Myocardial infarction among current OC users was four- to five times higher in women of Europe and developing countries, but this included women who also smoked and were hypertensive. The absolute risk in non-smoking women younger than age 35 was quite low—only 3 per million women-years. Several studies done in this country, including the Nurses' Health Study and the Kaiser Permanente Medical Care Program in California, indicate that oral contraceptives do *not* increase the risk of heart attack in women with no cardiovascular disease risk factors.

Guidelines for the use of oral contraceptives were published in the *Journal of Obstetrics and Gynecology* in 1993 to ensure safety from heart disease. Essentially, women over 35 who smoke or have elevated LDL-C with zero or one other risk factor for heart disease and stroke should not use oral contraceptives. More specifically, these guidelines are as follows:

Oral contraceptives may increase blood lipids, especially in women over age 35, women who smoke, or women with one or more risk factors for heart disease and stroke.

Women with known risk factors for heart disease and stroke should not use oral contraceptives.

❤ If LDL-C is less than 130 mg/dL, OCs can be used.

❤ If LDL-C is between 130 and 160 mg/dL, OCs can be used, but diet therapy to reduce saturated fat and cholesterol intake is needed.

❤ Women over 35, with two or more risk factors, should not use oral contraceptives.

❤ Women less than 35, whose LDL-C is between 160 and 190 mg/dL, and who have no more than one risk factor for heart disease, can use oral contraceptives in conjunction with diet therapy to reduce saturated fat and cholesterol intake.

❤ If LDL-C exceeds 160 mg/dL, and there are two or more risk factors present, oral contraceptives should not be used

Oral contraceptives and blood clotting

The relationship between oral contraceptives and blood clotting is probably the most important issue, and certainly, the most complex. The early oral contraceptive formulations appeared to cause thrombosis in some women. Some of these problems have persisted even with the low-dose formulations. The question of whether or not oral contraceptives cause stroke and *venous thromboembolism* remains an important—and controversial—issue.

Oral contraceptives—even the current low-dose formulations—increase your risk for venous thrombosis.

In the WHO study cited above, the risk of stroke increased nearly three-fold in European women who used oral contraceptives. But again, the odds were greatly reduced in women who did NOT smoke, were NOT hypertensive, and who used the lowest doses (<50 micrograms estradiol). The California based study, which included more than a million women, found that low-dose contraceptives did NOT increase risk of either hemorrhagic stroke or ischemic stroke. Smoking while using oral contraceptives greatly increases risk of hemorrhagic stroke.

The issue of *venous thromboembolism* has been more elusive. Recently, an inherited resistance to a specific clotting factor has been identified, and seems to be the basis for most cases of venous thrombosis in women who use oral contraceptives (as well as women who are pregnant). In the WHO study, risk of venous thromboembolism was three- to four-fold higher in OC users than nonusers. Unfortunately, the statistics do not yet justify routine screening for abnormalities in blood coagulation before prescribing oral contraceptives. Instead, physicians should inquire about your family history of thrombosis, and at the first sign of any circulatory abnormality with either contraception or pregnancy, you should seek genetic screening for blood clotting defects.

Risk of blood clot is higher in obese women and in those who are hypertensive. Smoking, in this case, does not seem to be a factor. And unfortunately, risk is not significantly reduced in women who use the newer low-dose oral contraceptive formulations. Death from venous thrombosis is about 14 per million users of low-dose OCs per year compared to only 5 per million non-users.

Other effects of oral contraceptives on cardiovascular factors

Although endogenous estrogen dilates blood vessels, apparently the artificial exogenous estrogens do not, because oral contraceptives increase blood pressure in most women. Although this rise in blood pressure probably does not require treatment, any woman who uses oral contraceptives should have a yearly blood pressure assessment by a qualified professional. This, of course, is particularly important if you have a history of hypertension, a strong family history of hypertension, or if your hypertension is controlled by medication.

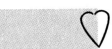

Oral contraceptives may increase insulin resistance and cause glucose intolerance in some women.

The risk for hypertension in users of oral contraceptives is considerably increased in those who smoke, are obese, or are over the age of 35.

Another potential problem is that of carbohydrate metabolism. Generally, oral contraceptives increase insulin resistance. The body adjusts to this by increasing the production of insulin with no change in glucose tolerance. However, some women will develop glucose intolerance and become hyperglycemic. Apparently, the progestin component of oral contraceptives is responsible for these changes in carbohydrate metabolism. The newest progestins have almost eliminated this effect, but women who are diabetic, or at high risk for diabetes should take special precautions, and especially women who had gestational diabetes with earlier pregnancy. There may be special risk of thrombosis in diabetic or glucose intolerant women who use oral contraceptives.

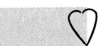

The new low-dose oral contraceptives carry a greatly reduced risk of heart disease and stroke compared to earlier formulations. But risk of venous thrombosis may remain.

In conclusion, I believe the evidence shows that the new low-dose oral contraceptive preparations carry a greatly reduced risk of heart disease and stroke than earlier formulations, but may still contribute significantly to risk of venous blood clot. Risks are considerably higher in women who smoke, are obese, hypertensive, or diabetic. In general, oral contraceptives are safe for women younger than 35 who have no risk factors for heart disease.

Risks are increased in women who are obese, smoke, hypertensive, or diabetic.

Postmenopausal Hormone Therapy

An overview

Postmenopausal estrogens are different from oral contraceptive estrogens.

First, they serve a different purpose. Contraceptive estrogens suppress the ovaries and prevent the production of endogenous estrogens. A strong, biologically active estrogen is needed to do this, and the artificial estrogens work quite well. In menopause, the natural production of estrogen by the ovaries has declined, and exogenous estrogen is used to supplement the estrogen your body still produces. Consequently, much less powerful estrogen is needed, and although the formulations of the many preparations differ, they are "conjugated estrogens," which are naturally produced from a horse (equine) or plant, rather than synthetic estrogens. These are often coupled with a mild form of synthetic progesterone, usually medroxyprogesterone acetate. Physicians prescribe the lowest dose that is sufficient to reduce menopausal symptoms. Obviously, with menopause there is no sense in suppressing whatever estrogen the ovaries remain capable of producing.

As explained earlier, estradiol is not the only form of estrogen a woman produces. As estradiol declines during the perimenopause, the estrogen that is produced by the adrenal glands and that is converted from adrenal androgen by body fat tissues, becomes dominant. This is known as *estrone*. The exogenous estradiol given for menopause supplements the endogenous estrone, and is used for three purposes. The first, and most widely known purpose, is the elimination of menopausal symptoms—hot flashes, vaginal dryness, and shrinkage of tissues in the breast and genital area. This is the usual reason women choose postmenopausal estrogen or hormone therapy. The second purpose, not so well known but perhaps of greater importance, is to reduce the loss of bone mineral and prevent the bone thinning that characterizes *postmenopausal osteoporosis*. Osteoporosis causes "dowager's hump," the stooped posture from progressive microfracturing of the thoracic spine, and the devastating hip fractures so common in old age. The third purpose for postmenopausal estrogen therapy is prevention of heart and vascular disease in old age. Many women are not aware of this benefit of postmenopausal hormone therapy—at least it is not a common reason for their choosing to use it.

Sounds good so far, right? If postmenopausal hormone therapy does all this for us, then why do so many woman choose not to use it? Remember the common expression "if something sounds too good to be true, it probably is?" Well, that may be the case here. Along with these wonderful benefits, postmenopausal hormone therapy carries some significant risks. The most prevalent risk is that of uterine cancer. Of course, this is not a problem for women with surgical menopause—their uterus was removed with hysterectomy. A secondary, and quite controversial risk, is that of breast cancer. The full story is quite complicated, but the following discussion should clarify it for you.

First, let's make sure you understand some terminology before continuing. *Postmenopausal estrogen therapy* refers to the use of oral (by pill) or transdermal (by skin patch) estrogen without the use of its antagonist, progesterone. This is called "unopposed estrogen." This regimen can be used by women who have had a hysterectomy because they have no risk of uterine cancer. It is *not* recommended for women with an intact uterus because unopposed estrogen stimulates the lining of the uterus (endometrium). A woman with an intact uterus who uses unopposed estrogen will eventually develop abnormally increased cellular growth (hyperplasia) of the endometrium, which if not shed (as in a menstrual period) may lead to significantly increased risk of uterine cancer. *Postmenopausal hormone therapy* refers to the use of oral or transdermal estrogen coupled with a progestin or progesterone that opposes the endometrial growth described above. Most often the progestin is added only during the last 10 days of each month. A woman who uses both postmenopausal estrogen and progesterone will usually resume or continue to have menstrual periods for a while—as long as her ovaries are still capable of producing a little estradiol. Eventually, her periods stop altogether.

So much for my quick overview. Let's look in more detail, first at the benefits of postmenopausal estrogen/hormone therapy, and then at the risks. Exactly what do these hormones do for us?

The benefits of postmenopausal hormones

<u>Menopausal symptoms</u>. It is well established that prescription postmenopausal hormones eliminate or considerably diminish menopausal symptoms. Hot flashes and the accompanying insomnia, irritability and depression are eliminated completely or greatly reduced. Hormone therapy reduces symptoms of vaginal and urinary tract atrophy (a wasting away or thinning of cellular tissues), and stress incontinence (inability to control urination with coughing, laughing or exercise). Vaginal walls retain (or regain) the ability to produce lubricating secretions in response to sexual arousal. This leads to increased comfort with sexual intercourse, and consequently, improved interest in sexual activity. Most everyone wants that, right? Postmenopausal estrogen increases blood flow to the brain and often improves short-term memory, mood, and cognitive function. No more locking yourself out of the house! Although claimed by the pharmaceutical companies, however, there is no evidence that postmenopausal estrogen decreases wrinkles or gray hair as many women believe. So, don't expect miracles with postmenopausal hormones. Nevertheless, most women report enhanced health and feelings of physical and psychological well-being while using postmenopausal hormones, either estrogen alone or estrogen plus progestin.

Physicians typically prescribe estrogen or estrogen plus progestin at as low a dose as will adequately reduce menopausal symptoms. This is usually 0.625 mg/day of conjugated estrogen (most often Premarin), and the progestin with the least negative effects, which in the United States is medroxyprogesterone acetate (Provera is the most common).

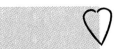

Postmenopausal estrogen or hormone therapy effectively reduces the menopausal symptoms:

- **Hot flashes**
- **Vaginal and urinary tract atrophy**
- **Shrinkage of breast and genital tissues**

It is also effective in protecting our bones. Postmenopausal estrogen improves our ability to absorb calcium from the foods we eat and the calicum sup-plements we take. It also stimulates our bones to increase the uptake of minerals when we do weight-bearing exercise.

Reduction of bone mineral loss. Osteoporosis is the severe thinning of our bones that results from progressive loss of mineral from the interior of our long bones and spine. The process of bone mineral loss, which begins sometime in our late thirties and is accelerated at menopause when our production of endogenous estrogen declines dramatically, causes at least 250,000 hip fractures and 500,000 spinal microfractures per year. Hip fracture usually leads to loss of physical independence, and often to admittance to a nursing home. It is frequently a devastating disability. Spinal microfractures initially cause a loss of height, and eventually, the unsightly and disabling dowager's hump.

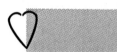

Oral postmeno-pausal estrogen lowers total cholesterol, decreases LDL-C, and increases HDL-C, offering significant protection from heart disease to postmenopausal women.

Adding progestin in the form of medroxyprogest-erone acetate or micronized progesterone does not significantly alter these benefits.

Although increased calcium consumption and weight-bearing exercise is advocated for reduction of bone mineral loss, estrogen is essential for maximal results. Without exogenous estrogen during menopause, our intestines fail to absorb much of the calcium we consume whether it is in the food we eat or the calcium supplements we take. Many studies have shown that although bones respond in a positive way to the stresses placed upon them with weight-bearing exercise, the response is considerably increased when we also consume exogenous estrogen. In scientific jargon we say "calcium consumption (supplementation) and weight-bearing exercise are most effective *in the presence of estrogen.*" That means we receive little benefit from the calcium we consume and the weight-bearing exercise we do if we do not also receive postmenopausal estrogen.

As I mentioned, the best documented benefit of postmenopausal estrogen therapy is prevention of osteoporosis.

Effects on blood lipids. The oral estrogens—conjugated estrogen or estradiol—significantly alter the blood lipids of postmenopausal women for the better, particularly in those who have high cholesterol. Total cholesterol decreases, LDL-C decreases (about 4%) and HDL-C increases (about 10%); the extent of the changes depends largely on the initial levels. The worse they are initially, the better the responses to the postmenopausal estrogen. The triglyceride content of both HDL-C and LDL-C increases with postmenopausal estrogen. One study reported huge changes in women with initially high blood lipids who also followed a stringent, low-fat anti-atherosclerosis diet. There was a 13% reduction in cholesterol, a 27% reduction in LDL-°C, a 24% increase in HDL-C, and a 30% increase in triglyceride. These lipid changes would decrease risk of cardiovascular disease by 50%. Wow!

Adding a progestin is problematic because progestins tend to be androgenic, which means that they produce male characteristics including blood lipid changes that increase the risk of atherosclerosis. But the effects of progestins on blood lipids depend on the type and dose used. For years, adding a progestin to postmenopausal estrogen therapy was thought to nullify the beneficial effects of estrogen on blood lipids. The Postmenopausal Estrogen/Progestin Interventions (PEPI) study has changed that thinking.

The PEPI Trial was completed in 1995. This very important and well-conducted research studied the effects of conjugated estrogen alone, and in combination with three different progestins and prescription regimes, on changes in blood lipids. The results showed that in women with a uterus, conjugated estrogen with medroxyprogesterone acetate or micronized progesterone (like a time-released progesterone) added in the last 10 days resulted in beneficial effects nearly identical to those produced from using conjugated estrogen alone. This means that the progestins with the least tendency to enhance atherosclerosis are medroxyprogesterone acetate and micronized progesterone. Unfortunately, micronized progesterone is hard to get.

Many women today are using the estrogen skin patch. With the skin patch, estrogen is absorbed directly into the blood—it is not first routed to the liver as is oral estrogen that must pass through the digestive tract. This may reduce risk of liver cancer and improve the absorption of estrogen because it does not first have to be absorbed by the intestine as it does in pill form. However, the jury is still out on whether transdermal postmenopausal estrogen is as effective as oral estrogen relative to the blood lipids.

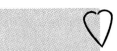

Unlike the oral contraceptives, postmenopausal estrogens do *not* increase the tendency of blood to clot. In fact, menopausal hormone therapy reduces the tend-ency for blood to clot, and once formed, enhances clot busting. Thus, hormone therapy adds to its pro-tective effect re-lative to heart and vascular disease.

Effects on blood clotting. The less biologically powerful postmenopausal estrogens do NOT cause the problems with blood clotting that are found with the stronger oral contraceptive estrogens. Postmenopausal estrogen reduces the tendency of blood to clot by lowering the concentration of a substance in blood called *fibrinogen*, which plays a major role in clotting. This is beneficial for prevention of heart and vascular diseases in middle-aged and older women. Again, the PEPI study confirmed that fibrinogen increases during menopause when there is no hormone therapy, but that conjugated estrogen taken alone or coupled with a progestin lowers fibrinogen and contributes to the protective effect of postmenopausal hormone therapy with respect to heart disease and stroke.

A recent study indicates that postmenopausal hormone therapy actually helps break up blood clots—that is, it is a "clot buster." Thus menopausal hormone therapy not only prevents clots from forming, but hastens their removal when they do form. This, then is still another mechanism whereby hormone therapy protects postmenopausal women from heart disease.

Other effects of postmenopausal hormones. As explained earlier, insulin resistance and impaired glucose tolerance are important factors in the development of heart disease in women. Estradiol, the dominant form of premenopausal estrogen, improves insulin sensitivity, but most early formulations of progestin did the opposite causing insulin resistance. So the question for many years was—what happens when postmenopausal women use conjugated estrogen therapy coupled with the newer non-androgenic progestin formulations? We now have the answer from several studies conducted in the 90s (including the PEPI study), and it is good

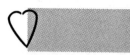

Current research clearly shows a significant reduction in heart disease, heart attack, and death in postmenopausal women who use hormone therapy

news. They do not counteract the estradiol-induced improvement in insulin sensitivity.

Postmenopausal hormones also were questioned because of the association between hypertension and the earlier high-dose oral contraceptives. Good news again! Major studies show no adverse effects of postmenopausal hormone therapy on blood pressure—in either women with normal blood pressure or hypertension.

Reduction in heart disease. Many studies have shown a significant reduction in risk of heart disease, heart attack and death in postmenopausal women using hormone therapy. It is estimated that overall reduction of risk may be as much as 50%, whether or not a woman has known risk factors for heart disease.

I've mentioned the Nurses' Health Study several times before. In 1991, it was reported that postmenopausal women in this on-going study who used conjugated estrogen had significantly reduced risk of heart disease, but not stroke, whether they had a natural or surgically induced menopause. An earlier report had shown that the protective effect was greatest in women who had had double oophorectomy. A 1996 follow-up of the Nurses' Health Study showed a 40% reduction in women who used estrogen alone, and a nearly 70% reduction (!) in women who used postmenopausal estrogen with progestin, but again, no reduction in risk of stroke. Based on these and other results, scientists proposed that postmenopausal estrogen be the standard of care in countries such as the United States where heart disease is the leading cause of death and a major cause of illness in women. This has created a lot of controversy because there is criticism of the interpretation of some of these results.

What's wrong—if anything—with all these data? The major criticism is that all these wonderful positive results come from studies that have what is called "_selection bias._" This means that the selection of subjects in the study may affect the outcome of the study. For a study to be objective, or unbiased, the subjects should be recruited from the general population. They should be assigned at random (by chance alone) to either an experimental group who receives the drug or treatment or to a control group who does not receive the drug or treatment. In this way, researchers can objectively compare the effects of the treatment. But in many studies, subjects were not randomly assigned to control or experimental groups. Rather, the women who already used postmenopausal hormones were assigned to the experimental groups, and the women who did not use hormones were assigned to the control group. This is important because women who use postmenopausal hormones are more likely to be upper-middle class, white, and well-educated (at least high school) than the average American woman. They are also more likely to watch their diets carefully, to exercise regularly, and to be leaner than those who do not use hormone therapy. These factors may cause yet another possible bias—compliance bias. Such women are more likely to comply correctly with instructions given by the investigators.

In addition, doctors are less likely to give hormones to women with known heart disease, high blood pressure, and diabetes for fear that they may experience blood clots. And so the women in the experimental groups are unusually healthy women. All these factors contribute to selection bias. So the question is: could these wonderfully positive results merely be "a healthy woman effect?"

The "healthy women selection bias" was strikingly demonstrated by the Healthy Women's Study in 1996. This study followed 355 premeno-pausal women through menopause. The researchers showed that the women (mostly white) who chose to take postmenopausal hormones had more favorable levels of HDL-C, blood pressure, fasting insulin, body weight, physical activity and alcohol intake than the women who did not do so. They were also more highly educated.

The bottom line is that the benefits of postmenopausal hormone therapy relative to protection from heart disease are likely to be exaggerated, and the risks minimized. Dr. Andrew Weil points out that if you take women who are not likely to develop heart disease, put them on a drug—and remember, postmenopausal hormone therapy is a drug—they are still unlikely to develop heart disease. If they "get" anything, it is going to be something else—and so the risk of cancer relative to the risk of heart disease may be overstated.

Let's look at that risk now.

The risks of postmenopausal hormone therapy

We've discussed the benefits of hormone therapy at menopause quite extensively. If that was the "rest of the story" women would be flocking to physicians for prescriptions. But they aren't. There is a hesitancy not only on their parts, but on the part of many of their physicians. Why the worry? In a word—cancer.

Uterine cancer. The history of postmenopausal estrogen use, although scary, is helpful. In the 1960s, a best-selling book (_Feminine Forever_) argued that menopausal women treat estrogen deficiency or become sex-less, unattractive old hags. The book, written by a male physician, was a sensation, and millions of women flocked to their doctors for this fountain of youth known as "estrogen replacement therapy." Following the urging of the pharmaceutical companies, physicians prescribed postmenopausal hormones to millions of women. (Note that in all my discussion of meno-pause I have not used the phrases "estrogen deficiency" or "estrogen replacement." That's because the more modern view of menopause is that it is not a disease, that there is nothing wrong with you when you have menopause, and that there is not a deficiency of anything. Rather, menopause is a natural lessening of ovarian function that happens to all women when their child-bearing years are over. Back to our story.)

Well, guess what? An epidemic of uterine cancer followed. Women taking the estrogen replacement regimes of the 60s and early 70s developed uterine cancer at a rate six times higher than women who ignored all the hype, and did not use estrogen at all. Naturally, the popularity of estrogen therapy plummeted. It has still not completely recovered.

Of course medical scientists did not sit still during all this, and with considerable financial support from the drug companies, went to work to find out what had gone wrong. This flurry of research resulted in significant breakthroughs in the formulations of exogenous estrogens. They found that different types of estrogen had different actions on the body. Conjugated "natural" estrogens (from pregnant mare's urine or from plant sources—soybeans, mostly) were found to have less powerful actions than the synthetic estrogens needed for contraception. In the 1980s, we learned that very low-doses were sufficient to reduce or eliminate menopausal symptoms, and a whole new generation of estrogen and progestin formulations were developed for "treatment" of menopause.

My mention of progestin is significant. Remember that progesterone is an antagonist to estrogen because some of its actions oppose those of estrogen. It was found that adding a form of progestin to estrogen therapy prevented the *endometrial hyperplasia* (abnormal cellular growth) that is the precursor of uterine cancer. Now, since the 80s, physicians recommend "hormone therapy"—the combination of low-dose estrogen and a mild progestin. The result is that risk of uterine cancer with such a regimen has been greatly reduced—but the risk is still not zero.

Part of the PEPI study examined the effects of estrogen taken alone and estrogen with progestin on the endometrial tissues of postmenopausal women. The major strength of this study was that the subjects were randomly assigned to receive one of five different regimens. This eliminates nearly all of the selection bias that occurred in many other studies of the effects of postmenopausal hormone therapy on heart disease. The regimens used in PEPI were placebo (an inert substance—i.e., a fake), conjugated equine estrogen taken alone, and three regimens of estrogen taken with a progestin. A weakness of the study was that nearly all the subjects were white (only 4% were African Americans and 3% were Hispanic).

The results confirmed that a daily dose of 0.625 mg (the commonly used low-dose) of conjugated estrogen, taken alone, may result in endometrial hyperplasia. Over 34% of the women on this regimen developed some form of endometrial hyperplasia. The women given any of the estrogen plus progestin regimens had no more hyperplasia than those taking the placebo. This confirms that combining low-dose conjugated estrogen with medroxyprogesterone acetate or micronized progesterone protects the endometrium from hyperplastic changes that occur when es-

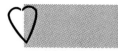

The use of post-menopausal estrogen without progestin or progesterone will increase the risk of uterine cancer in a woman with an intact uterus.

trogen is taken alone. Obviously, any menopausal woman with a uterus who is taking estrogen should also be using a progestin, and if she is not, should be screened for uterine hyperplasia every year.

Well what about breast cancer? This is even more complicated.

Breast cancer. Like the uterus, breast tissue also responds to exogenous estrogen, so it was logical for investigators to examine the relationship between postmenopausal estrogen and the incidence of breast cancer. The results of these investigations seem to be conflicting. Only in recent years has additional light been shed on this complicated and serious question.

Initial evidence was from studies in which animals were given exogenous estrogens. The animals (mostly mice) developed mammary tumors that grew rapidly. Similarly, human breast cells exposed to exogenous estrogen in the laboratory often became malignant. But, results from population-based studies of women using postmenopausal estrogen were mixed. Most showed no increase in breast cancer, or very minute increases. A few studies even showed less breast cancer in women using postmenopausal estrogen.

The problem with many of these studies was that among the subjects were women who had answered "yes" to such questions as "have you ever used postmenopausal estrogen?" or " have you used postmenopausal estrogen at any time?" This means that women who had used estrogen therapy for as little as a month or two, or had used hormones off and on, were included as subjects, as well as women who had used hormones for quite some time. No wonder the confused results.

I've studied this issue thoroughly because I have used postmenopausal estrogen since the age of 41 following a hysterectomy and double oophorectomy. At age 57, I was diagnosed with intraductal carcinoma in situ (the good news was that this is a noninvasive, very early stage cancer). So I've given very careful thought to the risk of breast cancer and postmenopausal estrogen therapy. I've read practically all the studies and the best summary appears in the World Health Organization's Technical Report Series #866, _Research on the Menopause in the 1990s_, which I paraphrase here. The authors of this report carefully analyzed the conflicting information relative to "duration of use" of exogenous estrogen. They concluded that:

- ❤ the use of postmenopausal estrogens for less than 5 years does not increase risk of breast cancer,
- ❤ use of estrogens for 5 to 9 years may result in a "small" increase in risk of breast cancer, but results are highly variable
- ❤ use of estrogens for 10 or more years may be associated with a 30 to 80% increase in risk of breast cancer,
- ❤ the addition of progestins in combination with postmenopausal estrogen is not yet clear, but most likely does not reduce the risks outlined above.

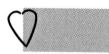

The use of post-menopausal hormone therapy does not increase risk of breast cancer if used for less than five years. Long term use—10 years or more—may significantly increase risk of breast cancer.

An interesting study was recently published on mortality among women in the Nurses' Health Study. Among the women who used postmenopausal hormones, mortality was 37% lower compared with those who did not. Most of this was due to a low number of deaths from heart disease, but the results also showed a high rate of death from breast cancer in women who had taken hormones for more than 10 years. So menopausal hormone therapy protects you from heart disease, but the survival benefits diminish the longer you use it.

It is obvious that a woman who uses menopausal estrogen or hormone therapy should be screened regularly—once per year—for breast cancer. Although mammography is good at that, it does not detect every instance of breast cancer.

The risk-benefit ratio

So what's a postmenopausal woman to do? If she chooses to use estrogen or hormone therapy she may decrease her risk of heart disease by as much as 50%, and significantly reduce her bone mineral loss and risk of osteoporotic fractures in her spine and hip. But at the same time she may increase her risk of uterine or breast cancer. It is obviously a question of comparing your risks for heart disease and osteoporosis with your risks for uterine and breast cancer. This is known as a risk-benefit ratio—and it is something that every women, most likely with the help of a healthcare professional, needs to do.

It begins with an assessment of your risks for heart disease, osteoporosis, and cancer. Chapter 4 dealt with assessment of your risk for heart disease. This was quite complete, and speaks for itself. Complete assessment of your risks for osteoporosis and cancer is beyond the scope of this book so I'll be brief.

- ❤ If you have a family history of either of these diseases, you are at risk.
- ❤ If you are sedentary, you are at risk for osteoporosis.
- ❤ If you are overweight, your risk of osteoporosis may be less (because you stress your bones simply by standing on them), but your risk of breast cancer may be elevated because the more body fat you have, the more estrone you produce.
- ❤ If you drink a lot of coffee or cola drinks, and you do not drink much milk or eat much yogurt or dark green leafy vegetables, your calcium consumption is probably low, and you are at risk for osteoporosis.
- ❤ If you had an early menopause, have not had a child, or had a child after age 30, you are at increased risk of breast cancer.

In general, women have an almost 32% chance of dying of heart disease, compared to only a 2.8% chance of dying of breast cancer, and a 2.8% chance of dying from the complications of hip fracture. But remember that group statistics do not necessarily predict what happens to individuals. If you are at high risk for heart and blood vessel disease and at low risk for breast cancer, the benefits of hormone therapy outweigh the risks. On the other hand, if you are at low risk of heart and vascular disease and high risk for breast cancer, the benefits may not outweigh the risks.

I think you get the picture. You need to weigh the expected benefits of menopausal hormone therapy in terms of your risks for heart disease and osteoporosis, relative to your possible risks for uterine or breast cancer.

You also need to weigh your subjective feelings and emotions about use of estrogen/hormone therapy. Perhaps you don't want to take any risks. You fear cancer and don't want to take any chances whatsoever. Only you can determine that. And you need to respect whatever feelings you have about the matter. These feelings are not silly.

But estrogen therapy is not the only alternative a woman has. As stated in earlier chapters, heart disease is largely a disease of lifestyle. The following chapters describe lifestyle modifications that will reduce your risk of heart disease whether you choose to use postmenopausal hormone therapy or not.

Introduction to Part II:
Heart Healthy Habits

Part I was pretty grim, wasn't it? You learned a lot about heart disease, the risk factors for heart disease, and yourself relative to those risk factors. You learned that more women die of heart disease than any other chronic illness and that you or a loved one may well be at risk for a heart attack (or a second heart attack). Well, you can change that.

Part II of *Healthy Hearts, Healthy Women* provides the means, the "how-to," for making important lifestyle changes that will lower your risk of heart disease (or heart attack if you already have heart disease) and reverse many of the signs and symptoms you currently have.

Part II is a comprehensive approach aimed at altering some of the fundamental lifestyle causes of heart disease. Anything less than this would only provide temporary relief, and the physical manifestations, symptoms and problems associated with heart and vascular disease, would most likely recur. For example, coronary by-pass surgery clearly improves blood flow to cardiac tissues, and so too, does angioplasty (see Appendix B). But if you do nothing else, those vessels will re-clog or additional cardiac vessels will become occluded. Often within as little as six months time you are likely to be right back where you were before surgery. In other instances, surgery or other purely "medical" treatments may actually contribute to the development of new problems—stroke, infection, chronic obstructive pulmonary disease (COPD). An approach that simply treats symptoms, as is the case with solely drug or surgical treatments, and not fundamental lifestyle change, is temporary at best. Often one set of problems is merely traded for another. According to Dr. Dean Ornish, it is like applying a "physiological band-aid". Working at a deeper level to avoid or reverse heart disease is absolutely essential. Part II of this book provides a comprehensive program for adopting lifelong heart healthy habits—nothing less will work. Closely following this program will reduce your risk of heart and vascular disease. If you have been told you have heart disease or if you have already had a heart attack, following this program may reverse your disease. Be sure to tell your doctor about your intention to follow this program before you begin so that any individualized adjustments can be made. Coupled with good medical care, Heart Healthy Habits will give you a new lease on life. Here's a bird's eye view of that program.

WHAT'S TO COME IN PART II:
DEVELOPING HEART HEALTHY HABITS

Of greatest importance is daily heart healthy physical activity. Chapter 7, "Exercise: Essential for Your Heart," emphasizes the benefits of daily physical activity, describes what aerobic exercise is, why it is so important, and how you can easily and regularly "just do it." The chapter focuses on walking—an aerobic form of exercise that almost everyone can do, and guides you through developing an individualized program that begins easily and steadily progresses so that you will get the greatest possible benefit. You'll learn a very simple way to find the exercise intensity that is right for you. A walking technique is described that allows you to achieve fitness, avoid injury, and have fun while doing it. The chapter also includes straight-forward and practical tips for buying the right shoes, and care of your busy walking feet.

You will gain the most from daily physical activity when you also "eat right." And so, Chapter 8, "Eating for Your Heart," guides you to heart healthy eating habits that are nutritious and delicious!, and will allow you to lower your blood cholesterol, your blood pressure, lose weight if desired, and provide plenty of energy for your daily exercise efforts. You'll eat well, believe me! Although menus and recipes are not provided—because there are many excellent books that already do that and because you'll learn more when you do that on your own—this chapter will increase your food awareness, in fact, that is the primary goal of the chapter. Although there is plenty of material here, it is not complicated, and it is well worth every bit of the effort you put forth to learn the basic principles of heart healthy eating.

A lifestyle approach to altering your risk of heart and vascular disease would not be complete without addressing the nemesis of many women—stress. The mind-body connection is very strong and certainly not to be denied. Chapter 9, "De-stressing Your Heart," describes the stress response, both acute (sudden) stress and chronic (long-lasting) stress, and how they contribute to heart and vascular disease. The probable cause of most stress in women is described and the means to combat this cause are given. Following the lead of several highly successful programs for reversing heart disease and other chronic conditions (programs designed and conducted by Dr. Herbert Benson, Dr. Dean Ornish, Dr. Jon Kabot-Zinn), the emphasis in Chapter 9 is on combating stress by invoking opposing responses of pleasure and relaxation through simple breathing and meditation techniques that develop mindfulness and lovingkindness

Developing a health healthy lifestyle will:
  a) lower your risk of heart and vascular disease,
  b) prevent a second heart attack if you've already had one,
  c) improve your quality of life (even if you think you are healthy and happy now), and
  d) get you in better touch with your physical self.

You'll ultimately love these Heart Healthy Habits because they will make you feel better, look better, help you get in better touch with yourself, and raise your self-esteem. When you develop these Heart Healthy Habits you'll know that you are helping yourself because you are taking charge of your health—and ultimately, your life.

CHAPTER 6

Change:
Making the Commitment

A thousand mile journey begins with the first step.
—Lao-Tzu

Dr. Dean Ornish has proven rather substantially that you can actually reverse heart and vascular disease by adopting heart healthy habits. But, it takes effort, it takes commitment, it takes desire, it takes time—and it means making major lifestyle changes. You or any loved one, with heart disease or at risk of heart disease, can do it,

    if...you believe you can,

    if...you have sufficient desire to improve your health,

    if...you love yourself enough to really want to change.

Oprah Winfrey states in *Making the Connection*, "The most important part to understand [is] that it's...about making the connection. That means looking after yourself every day and putting forth your best effort to love yourself enough to do what's best for you."

Writing about her efforts to lose weight, she continues, "...it comes from the realization that taking care of my body and my health is really one of the greatest kinds of love I can give myself. Every day I put forth the effort to take care of myself, and there's no question I'm living a better life."

TAKING CHARGE OF YOUR HEALTH

It's time to take charge of your health and to change heart damaging habits. But changing your habits and behaviors—your sedentary lifestyle, the way you eat, and the way you cope with stress—isn't always easy. In fact, change of any kind can be difficult.

If you really want to change you have to change your perceptions of yourself, and especially your perceptions of yourself relative to the rest of the world. Unfortunately, we assume that the way we see things is the way they really are (or at least the way they should be). And, of course, if you really think about it, that is simply not true. According to Stephen Covey, author of the bestselling book *The Seven Habits of Highly Effective People*, "we see the world, not as *it is*, but as *we are*." (italics added) (p.28) And so, to change, you need to change how you are because real change comes from inside. According to Covey, making a change in your life requires that you have a sense of worth and security that comes from within, and is not dependent upon being liked by others, being treated well by others, having the attention of others, or being dealt all the "right" things or conditions in life. Further, making a change in your life requires that you be proactive— which means that you act independently of others and independently of circumstances—that you are self-reliant, rather than reactive and dependent upon others for your sense of worth.

Change Requires Being Proactive

Being *proactive* means that you are responsible for your own life, that you recognize that your behavior is a function of your individual decisions. Being proactive requires self-mastery.

People who are *reactive* do not score high on self-mastery. I'll use Covey's model to more clearly describe how being reactive is opposed to being proactive. The table below presents the conversational language and self-talk of reactive and proactive persons. A reactive person's language serves to shift responsibility away from themselves. It basically says, I am not responsible, someone or something outside of my control is responsible, and I can't do anything about it. It places blame elsewhere. The proactive person's language acknowledges cause or responsibility in the matter. By doing so, the proactive person recognizes that her behavior is at least partially responsible for the situation or condition she is in. The proactive person recognizes that she is independent as opposed to dependent upon someone or something else to determine how things will be or are. By doing so, she accepts responsibility for the way things are for her.

REACTIVE LANGUAGE	PROACTIVE LANGUAGE
There's nothing I can do about it.	Let's look at the alternatives.
That's just the way I am.	I can choose a different way.
He makes me so mad.	I control my own feelings.
I have to...(do something).	I will choose...(to do that or not).
I can't.	I will choose to .. or not.
I have to...	I prefer to...
If only..., then...	I will...

(from Covey, p.78)

The consequence of reactive language or self-talk is that it is self-fulfilling. For example, if you think you can't do something, whether that thought is right or not, you can't. And most likely that is because you don't even try. Reactive people are victimized because they do not take charge of their lives. In the case of heart disease and its risk factors, they think they have been dealt a nasty blow from the outside…"My father had heart disease, it runs in the family." "I've always been fat, it's just the way I am." "I've never been good at physical things, I'll never be able to follow an exercise program." "My body craves fats (or sweets), I'll never be able to change my diet." "I've always been the nervous type, I'm just not a calm person." These examples of reactive language place the blame or responsibility elsewhere; they deny *cause* in the issue and reject the possibility of change.

Being proactive, on the other hand, acknowledges independence. It is the "I can do it" attitude. "I am responsible." "I am self-reliant." "I can choose to (do it)…or not." "No one else is to blame for this but me." "I can change." Being proactive means that you take responsibility for yourself, and that you acknowledge that your behavior is a function of your decisions.

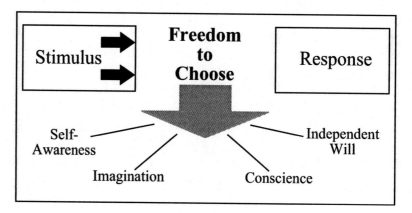

FIGURE 6.1
Proactive Model
(Reprinted with the permission of Simon & Schuster from *The Seven Habits of Highly Effective People*, p.71, by Stephen Covey. ©1989 Stephen R. Covey)

TO CHANGE, THE FIRST STEP IS DECIDING TO TAKE CHARGE.

YOUR FIRST STEP TOWARD CHANGE—SETTING REALISTIC GOALS

To begin, read Chapters 7, 8, and 9. Take some notes or write in the margins or use a highlighting marker so that you can go back to each chapter. Mark the things you do NOT currently include in your lifestyle, the things you need to pay special attention to, and all the behaviors, attitudes, and habits you need to change. You might also wish to mark—use a different color if you do this—all the heart healthy behaviors you already have, the things you have already incorporated into your life. After all, not everything is bad.

Then, considering what you need to change and what you already do, set goals—for exercise, for nutrition, and for stress release.

Goal setting is extremely important. By setting, and attaining goals, you exert personal control over your health and well-being. By setting goals, you chart your course toward a heart-healthy lifestyle. Without goals you will most likely flounder around aimlessly, moving from temporary change to temporary change without making any real *lifelong* changes. That is what you are after here. Remember, you are doing nothing less than changing your life to save your life. It is important to recognize exactly what is at stake here...your life.

But it is not quite that simple, goal setting is tricky. Goals must be *specific*, or you won't even know if you attain them. They must be *realistic*, or they won't be attained. They must be *personalized*, so that they are especially meaningful to you.

How do you go about setting specific and realistic and personalized goals? First, decide what your objective is—what it is you really want to achieve. It is improved fitness? Weight loss? Lower cholesterol? Reduced blood pressure (if you are hypertensive)? Improved glucose control? A less stressful and calm life? Most of these objectives, while admirable are pretty vague—they are not specific nor personalized, and depending upon circumstances, may not be realistic. But this is how you start.

Next, be specific about what you plan to do relative to each of these or other general objectives. For example, let's say that you have the objective of increasing your physical activity level. After reading Chapter 7, you decide to walk two miles on Mondays through Fridays each morning before going to work. That's what I mean by specific. This goal is specific and it is attainable. It specifies a particular behavior and when you are going to do it. Let's say that in addition, you want to take up a recreational sport for weekend activity. What sort of activity or sport really interests you? What sport will really sustain your longtime interest? What sport (or activity) will really give you pleasure over a long period of time? What sport will offer social incentives (if that is important to you)? Perhaps it is bicycling? swimming? hiking? canoeing? weight lifting at the gym? aerobics? tennis? Whatever sport or recreational activity you decide to take up, be specific about what you will do and how often you will do it. For example, let's say you decide to take up bicycling, and to go on one long ride each weekend. This is an example of setting a specific goal. You may need to go a step further and make specific interim goals—such as joining a local bike club, or finding a training coach to improve your cycling, or setting aside some money each week to buy a better bike. Get the idea?

For goals to work, they need to be specific. To establish specific goals ask yourself what? when? where? why?

For goals to work, they need to be realistic. What barriers are there to your success? Will you be able to pursue your chosen activity all winter? Will summer heat be a problem? Is the cost of equipment of gym membership prohibitive? The goals and resolutions provided in the following chapters are realistic for most people, but if you believe that they are not realistic for you—re-write them. By doing so, you will be personalizing these goals and resolutions.

For goals to work, you need to make them your own. Establishing goals to make someone else happy usually does not work. Establishing goals because you think you should usually does not work. Repeat three times—"I will not should on myself today." Goals must represent what *you* believe in, what *you* are interested in, what *you* deeply desire to attain. Otherwise you will lose interest, you will get bored, you will dislike what you are doing, and of course, you will ultimately fail.

After writing out your specific, realistic, and personalized goals, establish a timetable for accomplishment. Sometimes it is best to establish intermediate goals—with specific timelines for attainment of these intermediate goals. I'll use one of the heart healthy eating resolutions provided in Chapter 8 as an example. Suppose you have decided to accept the resolution to: eat at least 4 servings of legumes—beans, lentils, or peas—each week. Only, you have no idea about how to prepare legumes. Intermediate goals could be to buy a bean-based cook book (see RESOURCES section) and prepare one dish per week from that book. Another might be to buy a pressure cooker, learn how to use it, and prepare a large pot of beans every week. Perhaps you are not so sure you like legumes. An appropriate intermediate goal might be to add one legume-based dish to your usual cooking repertoire per week until you have found five legume-based recipes you really like and enjoy preparing on a regular basis.

BE POSITIVE

To achieve heart healthy habits you must set goals that are specific, realistic, and personalized.

Your attitude about changing lifelong habits is extremely important. Don't think only about "giving up things" (those delicious fatty foods, time in front of the TV set, etc) so that you can lower your cholesterol, reduce your blood pressure, or loss weight. Think instead of substituting better heart healthy behaviors for less heart healthy behaviors—like substituting low-fat cheese for full-fat cheese rather than eliminating all cheese, substituting cereal for eggs twice per week, learning how to avoid the "hidden fats" in cooking and omitting fried foods. Think about "healthy pleasures." As Drs. Robert Ornstein and David Sobel point out in their book *Healthy Pleasures*, that healthy habits need not be grim. It is not your goal here to live a deprived life—rather, your goal is to discover the "joie de vivre," the delight in a heart healthy life. You will soon discover that the healthiest people are pleasure-living, pleasure-seeking, pleasure-creating individuals who are not slaves to the work ethic. Think change, not sacrifice.

Cultivate an optimistic outlook, relish nature, enjoy a sauna or hot tub or massage, give hugs and enjoy touching, enjoy sex and have more of it, listen to music, enjoy good meals that are low in fat, enjoy the bounty of the land by eating more fruit and vegetables and grain-based foods, and above all—dance, both literally and figuratively. Dance the robust joy of life and health. Think of yourself as "born to be happy and healthy." Remember that it is the many small and often overlooked daily acts of life—even those that seem trite—that ultimately bring happiness.

ABOUT PROCRASTINATION

But I just don't have time" is the most common excuse (it is not a reason) for failing to adopt Heart Healthy Habits—especially daily physical activity. Of course you have time. Realize that you have simply chosen to NOT make time. You wouldn't think of leaving the house each day without brushing your teeth or combing your hair, or taking a bath—right? That's because your values dictate that you do that. You have chosen to brush your teeth and comb your hair each day because you believe that is a necessary part of being acceptable. You learned that. You have learned that nice, clean, acceptable people brush their teeth and comb their hair and you wish to be thought of as a nice, clean, and acceptable person. Now it is time to decide, that is, to make the conscious decision, that you will exercise every day. If brushing your teeth is important, shouldn't exercising your muscles, heart, and body be important too? I can't think of anything more important and I am not alone in believing that. More and more medical authorities who have previously ignored daily exercise as a form of disease prevention or treatment are agreeing that the number one thing everyone can do to prevent heart and vascular disease—is daily physical activity. So, why procrastinate? Of course you have time to exercise daily.

There are scores of books about time management, and nearly all of them point out that time management is about *values clarification*. Values are the rules or attitudes you have—conscious or unconscious—that guide your life. Your decisions about your behavior—whether you brush your teeth daily and exercise regularly—are based on your values. Some behaviors become lifelong habits you don't even think about any more (like brushing your teeth each morning). Other behaviors are based on conscious decisions you made every day (like whether or not to eat that donut, or whether you will walk before breakfast or before dinner).

If something seems to be in the way of accomplishing one of your goals, you need to examine this and consciously decide if that barrier is more or less important than your new goal. If you persistently put off working on one of your goals, you need to examine your feelings about that goal and what is getting in the way of accomplishing it. Identifying your feelings and discovering how you can get beyond the barrier is an important part of clarifying your values.

Of course you have time. You simply choose to make time.

Procrastination, itself, can be a major source of stress because you then berate yourself for failing to even get started. But sometimes the thought of facing the task you have set for yourself is so overwhelming, that you find yourself in a vicious cycle of procrastination, self-denigration, low self-esteem, and further procrastination. If you find yourself in such a situation, break up your original goal into tiny tasks, and do one at a time. Perhaps then, the goal will not seem so intimidating. For example, if walking every day for 30 minutes seems overwhelming to you, begin by walking 10 minutes. Then, as you find yourself adjusting to this, increase your walking time by 5 minute intervals until you have accomplished your goal of daily walking for 30 minutes.

Remember that life is time—a series of moments strung together. These moments create the pattern of your life. Defining your values to bring about lasting behavior change requires getting in touch with your inner feelings and clarifying your values about your health, your body, your diet, your way of life. Developing a loving relationship with yourself means loving your mind and your body—in balance. Loving yourself, not the withholding of love, motivates you toward health. Beginning to see your body as your friend and not as an enemy will take you a long way toward wanting to make changes in your lifestyle that will enhance your heart health. When you do that, the barriers to change will disappear. Believe me, it is well worth the effort required.

CHAPTER 7

Exercise:
Essential for Your Heart

Fitness is about living your life fully.
—James Rippe, M.D., Cardiologist

Daily exercise is the key to Heart Healthy Habits. This chapter will get you started on aerobic exercise that will be fun and easy to do, and yet will provide terrific benefits. It will make you feel better (even if you already feel well), it will enhance your feelings about yourself, and it will open up a whole new way of life for you.

Your Heart Healthy goal is

> *AT LEAST* 30 MINUTES
> OF MODERATE-INTENSITY AEROBIC EXERCISE
> MOST DAYS OF THE WEEK.

Think you'd heard that before? We are going to make it easy to accomplish this goal—something that might have seemed formidable to you before.

WHAT IS AEROBIC EXERCISE?

First of all, not just any kind of exercise will do; it must be aerobic exercise. So, what is *aerobic exercise*? It's simple really. To be aerobic:

- ❤ it must last at least 10 minutes
- ❤ it must involve the major muscle groups, and
- ❤ it must be rhythmic in nature.

Here's why. Aerobic means oxygen requiring. So an aerobic exercise is one that requires your body to produce energy via a process that *requires* oxygen. Think of this as a process that burns fuel in an oxygen flame. The advantage is that the aerobic process is capable of producing energy at a steady rate over a long period of time. The limiting factor is your ability to deliver oxygen to your muscles.

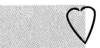

To be classified as an aerobic exercise, movement must:
- Be sustained at least 10 minutes
- Involve the major muscle groups
- Be rhythmic in nature

Good blood flow is necessary to deliver oxygen to your muscles and that is the role of your heart and vascular system. The heart pumps blood to tissues all over your body, but your muscles can also act as a pump that aids your heart. Alternating rhythmic contractions of large muscle groups actually help your heart deliver large quantities of blood—and oxygen— to your muscles for the aerobic production of energy. That's why walking, hiking, long-distance running (not sprinting), bicycling (not hill climbing), cross-country skiing, aerobic-dance (usually called "aerobics" at health clubs and spas), fancy ballroom dancing, and swimming are considered excellent forms of aerobic exercise. These alternating rhythmic muscular actions assist your heart in delivering blood and oxygen to your muscles so you do not tire quickly. In fact, when you have developed good cardio-vascular fitness—endurance fitness—you can perform these activities for long periods of time.

On the other hand, very sudden and/or powerful forms of exercise, like running up stairs or lifting a heavy weight, require another form of energy production—an *anaerobic* process. Anaerobic processes do not require oxygen to produce energy ("*an*" means not or without, so *anaerobic* means without oxygen). An anaerobic process is capable of producing energy very quickly (and that is its main advantage)—but you tire out rapidly, and have to stop. This is because anaerobic processes quickly use up the tiny amounts of fuel you have stored in your muscles, and produce acidic by-products that cause pain and fatigue. When you feel your muscles "burn," you are using anaerobic processes to produce energy. When your body relies on anaerobic metabolism, you will not be able to sustain activity very long at all.

To summarize this, aerobic exercise is fatigue resistant and can be sustained for long periods; anaerobic exercise is powerful but fatigue caus-ing, and can only be carried out for brief periods. It's rather like the old story about the tortoise and the hare. The tortoise relies on the steady production of a moderate rate of energy production—on aerobic pro-cesses—and never tires. The hare replies on the rapid production of en-ergy over short moments of time—on anaerobic processes—and tires quickly.

Of course it is not quite as simplistic as I've described. Most exercise is somewhat mixed—that is, energy is used that is produced both aerobi-cally and anaerobically. The point is that if you exercise at an intensity that exceeds your ability to deliver an adequate supply of oxygen to your muscles, then you are going to tire very quickly and you will have to slow down, or stop entirely. That is not aerobic exercise.

It is sustained exercise that will deliver all the benefits to be described shortly. It is aerobic exercise, that is particularly heart healthy. It is aerobic exercise that will enable you to lower your risk for heart and vascular disease.

Getting the picture? Aerobic exercise can be sustained as long as enough oxygen is delivered to your muscles. Using your major muscle groups in alternating, pumping-like actions—contract, relax, contract, relax—assist the heart in delivering the required oxygen. Voila! Aerobic exercise.

Many forms of exercise can be aerobic. The key is that there is no straining—as in weight lifting—and no explosive movements requiring sudden bursts of energy. Although any form of aerobic exercise is adequate for Heart Healthy Habits, I especially recommend walking because it is easy to do and assessable to everyone.

And so, your Heart Healthy goal is

> TO WALK BRISKLY AT LEAST
> 30 MINUTES MOST DAYS OF THE WEEK.

WHY WALKING?

Walking is the simplest and best form of exercise possible for your heart. Walking is the most natural form of all movements patterns we do. Humans are meant to walk. We have two legs, and we stand upright—we are designed to walk.

Walking is rhythmic. We swing our arms in coordination with our steps in a "cross-patterned" activity—as one leg swings forward, the opposite arm moves forward to counter the rotation of our pelvis. Apparently, the required electrical activity in the brain is very harmonizing and unifying, because there is something very soothing about walking and it can even be used to achieve deep meditation.

Walking obviously meets the three criteria above: it utilizes major muscle groups, it requires alternating rhythmic contractions of those muscles, and we can walk for long periods of time.

Before getting into the details of your Heart Healthy walking program, let's look at some very practical reasons that make walking such a wonderful activity. Walking has many advantages over other forms of exercise.

- ❤ You do not need to learn a new skill. Unless you have a disability that involves your lower extremities, you can walk.
- ❤ Walking does not require special equipment. All you need is a pair of well-fitting shoes that will cushion and support your feet.
- ❤ It costs nothing. You do not have to join a spa or get a personal trainer.

❤ You can do it anywhere—indoors or out-of-doors. I especially advocate outdoor walking because you will have contact with nature and I think that is important for your total physical as well as spiritual well-being. Being outdoors provides a sense of wholeness; of oneness with the universe that I believe is missing when walking indoors, but walking—is walking—and there may be times you prefer to walk indoors.

❤ The risk of injury is very small with walking, much less than running, swimming, or bicycling.

❤ Walking is not boring as is riding a stationary bike at home or spa.

❤ Walking can be a social activity (unlike swimming, for example). You can walk with friends, a fitness "buddy," family members, or your dog (and it's great exercise for the dog, too).

❤ And as I've already mentioned—you can enjoy the beauty and wholeness of nature while improving your fitness and helping your heart.

THE HEALTHFUL BENEFITS OF BRISK WALKING

Research confirms that daily brisk walking results in a number of physiological changes that are beneficial to your heart and general health. These benefits reduce your risk of heart disease and stroke, diabetes and glucose intolerance, obesity, and metabolic syndrome.

Daily brisk walking protects against the development of atherosclerosis by improving your blood lipid profile: (especially when coupled with the Heart Healthy diet described in Chapter 8.)

❤ it increases your HDL-C (the "good" cholesterol)
❤ it reduces your blood triglycerides
❤ it reduces your LDL-C (the "bad" cholesterol)
❤ it reduces your total cholesterol (TC)
❤ even if all these changes do not occur, your TC:HDL-C and/or LDL-C:HDL-C ratios will improve

Daily brisk walking protects against heart disease, peripheral vascular disease, and congestive heart failure:

❤ it protects against blood clots by decreasing blood platelet aggregation (platelet stickiness) and by increasing fibrinolysis (the breakdown of fibrin)

❤ it increases blood flow to the heart and blood distribution to the legs

❤ it increases the strength of the heart by directly enhancing the action of cardiac muscle. This improves heart function

Daily brisk walking protects against the development of hypertension and will decrease blood pressure if you are hypertensive:

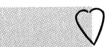

- ❤ numerous studies show that it reduces systolic and/or diastolic blood pressure in persons with high blood pressure.
- ❤ it decreases the amount of adrenalin in your blood. This allows blood vessels to relax and dilate. It also reduces the effects of emotional stress on your heart and blood vessels.
- ❤ with decreased blood pressure, the risk of stroke declines.

Daily brisk walking protects against the development of diabetes, insulin resistance, and obesity:

- ❤ it increases the sensitivity of muscle cells to insulin and thus improves carbohydrate metabolism. This prevents or reverses insulin resistance, and improves glucose tolerance.
- ❤ it uses body fat stores for energy and thus prevents weight gain and reduces obesity.

Daily brisk walking improves heart function in persons with hypertension or peripheral vascular disease, and in persons who have had a heart attack:

- ❤ it improves exercise tolerance, reduces fatigue, and reduces symptoms of cardiovascular disease.
- ❤ it reduces risk of illness and death in persons with heart and vascular disease. A recent study linked walking 4 hours per week with reduced risk of hospitalization and death from heart disease in elderly women (men, too).

Daily aerobic exercise such as brisk walking is heart healthy. There are many benefits:

- **It protects against atherosclerosis, hypertension, heart disease, peripheral vas-cular disease and con-gestive heart failure**
- **It improves your blood lipid profile**
- **It lowers blood pressure if ele-vated**
- **It improves insulin sensitivity and protects against diabetes and glu-cose intolerance**
- **It utilizes calories and uses body fat stores for energy, protecting against obesity**
- **It promotes strong heart function**

WHAT IS MODERATE-INTENSITY EXERCISE?

Exercise intensity is extremely important to achieve Heart Healthy goals. Strolling won't give you these benefits. Although you may achieve the social benefits, and it's relaxing, strolling will not increase your HDL-C nor alter the other factors mentioned above. Neither will exercising too strenuously. Harder and faster is not necessarily better. Exercising too strenuously will use anaerobic processes rather than aerobic processes, it may put strain on your heart, lead to unnecessary fatigue, and cause you to dislike exercise. You could also end up with an injury, and of course, that's self-defeating. So finding the RIGHT exercise intensity is very important.

I want to be very clear about this. The right exercise intensity is not one specific intensity for everybody. Rather, it is the right exercise intensity for YOU. This is to say that exercise intensity is always determined relative to your current physical fitness level. What is the right exercise intensity for you is likely to be too little for your daughter, and too much for your mother.

An excellent—but complicated way to determine you RIGHT exercise intensity level is to calculate your *target heart rate zone*. The method works, but quite frankly, the procedure is a "pain in the neck" and there is a much easier way. Nevertheless, I'm going to explain it, because it is important that you understand the basic principle of target heart rate zone. I'll explain the easier way shortly.

To determine your target heart rate zone, you must first estimate your *maximum heart rate*. This is the highest heart rate you can attain during a maximal exercise test. However, you don't have to actually do the test because it can be estimated by subtracting your age from 220 just about as accurately. For example: if you are 55, your maximum heart rate is 165 (220 minus 55 = 165). This is obviously much quicker and safer than completing a maximal exercise test. Besides, most people don't like to do them—they're exhausting!

Once your maximum heart rate is determined, then your target heart rate zone is determined by calculating 70% and 85% of that value. If you'd like to calculate your exact values, Appendix C (How to determine your target heart rate zone) will lead you through this calculation; but it is not really necessary because you can look at Figure 7.1 and determine these values closely enough. So do that now. Find your age at the bottom of Figure 7.1. Then read the numbers corresponding to the 70% and 85% maximum heart rate lines.

FIGURE 7.1
Target Heart Rate Intensity

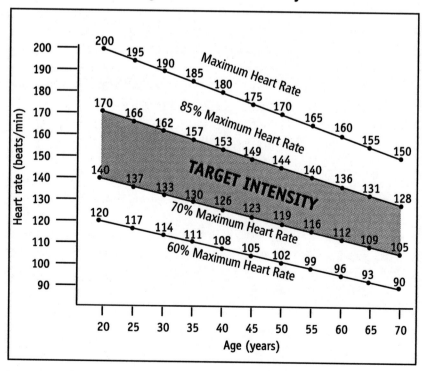

These numbers determine your target heart rate zone. Your job is to exercise within those limits because they signify your moderate-intensity exercise range. This is the right exercise intensity for you.

The 70% level reflects the minimum or lower level for achieving the Heart Healthy benefits described above. Exercising below this intensity will most likely not give you all the benefits you would like. The 85% level reflects the upper or maximum level for performing aerobic exercise. Beyond that level you are exercising too hard, you are performing strenuous exercise that has a major anaerobic component. Some athletes (but not all) need to train at that level to improve their performance, but you do not. Anaerobic exercise will not provide the Heart Healthy benefits described above—and in fact, could result in a serious strain on your heart. I repeat. The goal is to remain within the 70% to 85% target heart rate zone.

Unfortunately, this is where the "pain in the neck" part comes in. You have to keep taking your heart rate to see if you are within your target heart rate zone. Now if you'd like to do this, that's fine. A lot of people do, especially athletes who are seriously training to improve their performance. Their target heart rate zones are determined (usually at a higher level than are prescribed here), and they meticulously take their heart rates to be sure they are in their training zone. Some buy expensive heart rate monitors to do this. If you would like to use this method, I describe how to accurately take your heart rate in Appendix D (Measuring your heart rate) and estimated 10-second target heart rates in Appendix E (Target heart rate zones and...).

But I believe that most women don't really want to do this.

Exercising at your right TARGET INTENSITY is very important, but there is a much more enjoyable and less bothersome way to do this. It involves using your "feelings" (or perceptions) of exertion, and has been found to be very reliable and trustworthy. Being accurate is important, of course, but the best part of this is that it is so easy. This method is called *rating of perceived exertion.*

Moderate-intensity exercise is aerobic exercise. It will provide the heart healthy benefits you are aiming for.

Moderate-intensity exercise is achieved when you exercise within your target heart rate zone.

Your target heart rate zone represents 70% to 85% of your maximal heart rate.

RATING OF PERCEIVED EXERTION (RPE)

The basic principle is that your body is very smart and you simply need to listen to it and follow it's advice. RATING OF PERCEIVED EXERTION (RPE) is based on a subjective rating you identity in relation to specific "verbal descriptors." The RPE scale is related to your heart rate, your breathing, your metabolic rate, and various metabolic waste products in your blood. Therefore, it is closely related to the actual physiological stresses your body experiences.

To use the PERCEIVED EXERTION SCALE you simply rate your level of exertion using the descriptors on the scale below.

THE RATING OF PERCEIVED EXERTION SCALE		
RATING	DESCRIPTOR	
6		
7	Very, very light	
8		
9	Very light	
10		
11	Fairly light	
12		
13	Somewhat hard	*YOUR TARGET*
14		*INTENSITY*
15	Hard	
16		
17	Very hard	
18		
19	Very, very hard	
20		

You don't need to memorize the entire scale, or even carry a copy of it around with you. All you need to do is remember the following:

- the feeling of FAIRLY LIGHT Exertion is an RPE of 11
- the feeling of SOMEWHAT HARD Exertion is an RPE of 13
- the feeling of HARD Exertion is an RPE of 15

WHEN YOU EXERCISE BETWEEN THE PERCEIVED EXERTION LEVELS OF 13 TO 14 YOU ARE BETWEEN THE 70% AND 85% MAXIMUM HEART RATE LEVELS. YOU ARE AT YOUR TARGET INTENSITY.

Use rating of perceived exertion (RPE) to monitor your exercise intensity. Walking briskly at an RPE of 13 or 14 means you are at your target intensity for Heart Healthy benefits.

If your exertion level feels "HARD," that is, you are exercising at an RPE of 15, you are above your TARGET INTENSITY. This will lead to fatigue because your body is forced to use anaerobic metabolism. An RPE of 15 is about the upper limit for aerobic exercise, and consequently, for moderate-intensity exercise. Exercise at an RPE of 11 or below, and you are below the minimum intensity needed to sustain Heart Healthy benefits.

Another advantage of perceived exertion—besides its extreme simplicity—is that it can be used with any mode of exercise: brisk walking, lap swimming, road cycling, aerobic-dancing, cross-country skiing—including those in which obtaining an exercise heart rate is just not possible. It is appropriate for any form of "aerobic" exercise.

Best of all, perceived exertion is completely adaptable to your physical condition. As you become more and more fit, you will be able to walk at a faster rate while maintaining a perceived exertion of 13 or 14. So, once you are walking comfortably at an RPE of 13 or 14, you won't need to pay attention to your pace—it will take care of itself.

THE 60% MAXIMUM HEART RATE LEVEL

You will note above that Figure 7.1 also includes the 60% maximum heart rate level. For most people, this is below the minimum level for experiencing heart healthy benefits; but, there are many people for whom that statement is not entirely correct. If you have not exercised in many years, are overweight, currently have heart disease, high blood pressure, peripheral vascular disease, or angina with exertion, and if you have had a previous heart attack—this is where you should start. The 60% maximum heart rate level should be your goal until you and your physician are quite comfortable with your exercising at that level. This corresponds to a perceived exertion level of 12, somewhat more than FAIRLY LIGHT exertion (an RPE of 11). After a couple of weeks with no residual difficulties or problems of any kind, and when it is absolutely clear there is no unusual strain, discomfort, or cardiovascular symptoms of any kind, then you should move up into your TARGET INTENSITY at the 70% maximum heart rate threshold level.

If you have some form of heart or vascular disease (for example, hypertension or angina with exertion), you are overweight, or badly out of shape—begin exercising at 60% of your maximum heart rate. This corresponds to an RPE of 12.

When you and your physician determine that you are ready to do so, increase your exercise intensity to an RPE of 13 to achieve the full range of Heart Healthy benefits.

EXERCISE FREQUENCY—
WHAT IS MEANT BY "MOST DAYS OF THE WEEK?"

Go back to your heart healthy exercise goal for a moment:

> TO WALK BRISKLY AT LEAST 30 MINUTES
> MOST DAYS OF THE WEEK.

We've discussed exercise intensity rather thoroughly here because it is so important to achieve the results you want. But exercise frequency is also an important component of exercise prescription. Our stated goal includes the phrase "most days of the week." I've used this phrase because it is contained in exercise guidelines published by the National Institutes of Health, the American Heart Association, the American College of Sports Medicine, and the Surgeon General's Report on *Physical Activity and Health*, and it is quite appropriate here. You have probably already seen this phrase in media releases from the government, professional health organizations, HMO's, and health insurance companies. But it seems rather vague, doesn't it? Does it mean 4 days a week? 5 days a week? 6 days a week? 7 days a week? Four days represents more than half of seven—will that do?

The intent of the phrase was to indicate that people should exercise *every* day of the week (and sometimes the phrase "preferably all days of the week" is added), but while that is highly desirable, the writers of that policy felt there was also the need to provide some leeway. Stating that people should exercise every day of the week seemed arbitrary and rigid. Even the most well-intended person is likely to miss some days. Stating that you should exercise "most days of the week" allows you more freedom.

To achieve the Heart Healthy benefits of brisk walking, you should interpret the phrase "most days of the week" to mean at least five days a week. Assuming the expenditure of about 100 kilocalories for each mile walked, a sustained walk at about three miles per hour (that's 20 minutes per mile), will expend about 750 extra kilocalories per week if done five times per week for 30 minutes each time. This amount of energy expenditure has been consistently shown to yield the desired heart healthy benefits (reduction of total cholesterol, LDL-C and triglycerides, increase in HDL-C, reduction in elevated blood pressure, etc). If you walk seven times per week, this pace will expend about 1050 extra kilocalories per week, and the benefits will be even better.

I highly recommend that you walk briskly for at least 30 minutes every day of the week, but I also recognize that this is sometimes impossible to achieve, and occasionally, may not even be desirable. So—why not be reasonable about it?

EXERCISE DURATION—HOW LONG IS ENOUGH?

Well, I've covered exercise intensity and exercise frequency, and so to be complete, I should also discuss exercise duration. These are the three major components of an exercise prescription: some people like to use the acronym FIT for frequency, intensity, and time (duration).

Your goal is:

> TO WALK BRISKLY AT LEAST 30 MINUTES
> MOST DAYS OF THE WEEK.

There has been a flurry of research on exercise duration in recent years. A few years ago all exercise and fitness guidelines stated that 20 minutes of continuous exercise was the very least that would elicit fitness benefits. More recently, several studies have shown that separate 10 minute bouts of exercise—at the same intensity—that were spread throughout a day yielded about the same benefits if the total exercise time was 30 minutes. There are some practical advantages of three-10 minute exercise bouts per day compared to one-30 minute exercise bout. It is sometimes easier to find three uninterrupted 10 minute periods of time than it is to find a single uninterrupted 30 minute period. This is probably particularly true for women with small children (and maybe even big children). It may also be true for women who work—they could walk 10 minutes in the morning, 10 minutes at lunch (and still eat lunch), and 10 minutes in the evening. Personally, I prefer the single exercise period, and I continue to believe (but can not prove) that a single longer period is better than several short periods of exercise. But, again, the object here is to be flexible and not to impose an arbitrary and rigid exercise goal that few women can achieve. So although I would prefer that you exercise once a day for at least 30 minutes an exercise session, two or three shorter periods that total 30 minutes or more per day is OK too.

A RECOMMENDED ALTERNATE TO BRISK WALKING

You may not want to walk every day. If you're at all like me, you may thoroughly enjoy moving to music. I've already mentioned the "aerobics" that are done at fitness centers and health spas. Most often this is done to loud rock music with fully color-coordinated (sweat band to leg warmers) "instructors" gyrating vigorously and yelling out the moves in front of a class of sometimes as many as 50 people. If this appeals to you, great. Go for it! Apparently it appeals to many, because these classes always seem to be full.

It does not appeal to everyone, however, especially older women, women who are shy, women who are overweight, or women with limited fitness—and certainly there is not much individual attention in the type of situation I've described. It can be pretty daunting to attend such a class if you are a rank beginner at it.

What I've described is not at all what I mean when I advocate "aerobic-dancing" as an alternative to brisk walking. What I recommend is simply turning on your favorite CD or tape (the radio will also do)—and having a wonderful time doing your own dance or exercise movements to the music. Letting yourself go, being creative in your movements, being totally uninhibited in the privacy of your living room with no critics present to watch or judge you, and no worries about what others will think, can be a joyful and liberating experience. And, it is wonderful exercise. You can explore all the muscles of your body. You can swing your arms, leap, gyrate to your heart's content—and I mean that both figuratively and literally. You don't need an instructor, and you don't need a leotard with matching sweat band. Just let it all hang out. Just do it!

You may also want to try some exercise videos. Many are quite good, but beware of programs that are too vigorous for you. If, after watching a video through it doesn't appeal to you—don't use it.

BEFORE YOU BEGIN

Should You See Your Doctor Before Beginning?

The issue of medical clearance has been argued back and forth for decades. Formerly, it was recommended (probably because doctors and fitness specialists were afraid of malpractice suits) that everyone should obtain medical clearance before beginning an exercise program. If you really think about that it's pretty scary, isn't it? It implies that exercise is or could be dangerous. Well, we've learned better. There are very few negative health episodes resulting from exercise. Requiring medical clearance just filled doctor's appointment books and spent your hard-earned dollars.

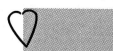

If you have known heart or vascular disease—you should consult your physician before beginning your brisk walking program.

Most adults do not need medical clearance or pretesting (an exercise stress test, for example) before beginning a moderate-intensity exercise program. However, anyone with known heart or vascular disease should seek medical clearance before beginning an exercise program. According to the National Institutes of Health, women over 50 with multiple risk factors for heart disease and stroke (but no known disease) should have a medical evaluation before starting a *vigorous* exercise program. This means that if you stay within your TARGET INTENSITY—which is moderate exercise—medical clearance is not necessary. However, if you have angina or undiagnosed chest pain with exertion, I strongly recommend that you consult your physician before beginning a regular program of brisk walking.

A number of years ago a very simple questionnaire was designed to help you evaluate your readiness to begin an exercise program. The PAR-Q (Physical Activity Readiness Questionnaire) helps identify the small number of people for whom physical activity may be inappropriate or who should seek medical advice concerning the type of activity most suitable for them. Common sense is your best guide to answering these few questions. Read the questions carefully, and check the yes or no space opposite the question as it applies to you.

Your Only Need—Walking Shoes

Get rid of your old sneakers, or relegate their use to shopping and housework. Your feet deserve good care. Begin to think like an athlete and that means using good equipment. One of the practical advantages I gave for walking was that you did not need equipment. And you don't. But you do need good shoes. Shoes designed for walking. Shoes you will use ONLY for walking. That will ensure that they will remain in good shape for a long time.

To get good walking shoes go to a sport shoe store and ask for their walking specialist (no, I'm not kidding). Discount stores are OK for price, but you won't get any special attention, and the salesclerk (if you can find

Yes	No	**PAR-Q AND YOU**
___	___	1. Has a doctor ever said that you have a heart condition and recommended only medically supervised activity?
___	___	2. Do you have chest pain brought on by physical activity?
___	___	3. Have you developed chest pain in the past month?
___	___	4. Do you tend to lose consciousness or fall over as a result of dizziness?
___	___	5. Do you have a bone or joint problem that could be aggravated by the proposed physical activity?
___	___	6. Has a doctor ever recommended medication for your blood pressure or a heart condition?
___	___	7. Are you aware through your own experience, or a doctor's advice, of any other physical reason against your exercising without medical supervision?

one at all) will not know very much about either the products available or your feet. Working with a sport store specialist will ensure that you end up with a good product, one that fits your needs, and you will get your money's worth.

There's a lot to know about sport shoes and the specific needs of each sport. That's why there are running shoes, walking shoes, aerobics shoes, basketball shoes, etc. All sports shoes are not the same. In walking, there is a heel-toe rocking motion with moderate impact at the heel followed by a transfer of weight to the ball of the foot for push-off. A good walking shoe will have a low heel, a reinforced heel counter to control the angle of the foot as it hits the ground, and a curved sole that supports your weight as it is transferred forward. Don't buy a cheap pair of general athletic shoes, they will not provide these features and you will be wasting your money. Expect to spend between $50 and $70.

I recommend trying on several brands because each has a certain "feel" to it, and is usually known for some feature. New Balance™, for example, has more variety in shoe widths than many others. Nike™ is known for its wide toe box. Asics™ is known for its softness and flexibility (which is fine unless you need more support). When you find a brand that fits you well and has a good "feel" you will probably want to stick with that brand for quite some time.

The single most important thing, of course, is fit. Besides not hurting your foot, what makes a good fit? You should have ¼ inch of space between your longest toe and the front of the shoe when standing on each leg. There should be no excessive movement of your heel in the heel cup or you're likely to get blisters. The lacing should be comfortable over your instep. The arch support should comfortably fit the natural curve of your foot. Be sure there isn't any stitching where your little toe is (a problem I often have) and that the toe box is right for your foot.

All you need are well fitting walking shoes, water-wicking socks, and loose fitting clothing. Go for it!

Your foot bends when you walk; and therefore, the shoe should flex easily. You want good foot support, but you don't want too stiff a shoe. Breathability is important too. If you live in a warm climate or your feet tend to sweat a lot, I recommend shoes of some mesh material. I personally find all-leather shoes too hot. Ask your walking shoe expert about the different materials. I also recommend light colored shoes because dark colors absorb heat from the sun and you may feel like your feet are baking.

Spend quite a bit of time getting your walking shoes. Don't do this hurriedly. A good shop expects you to take your time, to walk around the store quite a lot—they may even suggest you walk outside on the sidewalk or mall corridors so that you can stride out and feel what the shoe will do for you. A number of major sporting shoe stores even have "tracks" for you to try out shoes.

Socks are important too, so give them second thought. They should wick away sweat and protect against pressure points between your foot and shoe. Avoid cotton socks. Cotton absorbs moisture and stays wet. In cool weather, your feet will feel cold. I recommend the new acrylic-fiber blends. They are very soft, but best of all, they wick wetness away from your foot so that your foot stays dry. Wool socks are excellent for this as well, but they are hard to find and they shrink easily. Buy several pairs of different socks to try—no doubt you will find a particular brand, design, or fabric that will be just right for you.

What to Wear

You can be as plain or fancy as you want—but really, nearly anything will do. Some people like form-fitting leotards (that's what you see in all the glitzy fitness magazines), but I prefer loose fitting clothing that allows plenty of movement of both your legs and arms, but is not too bulky. Warm-up pants are great. So are shorts (when weather permits). There are some really attractive "sweats" available from Sears and Mervyn's that are very reasonable in cost. But you don't need to buy anything special. Your baggy old slacks will do in cool weather, your old bermuda shorts in warmer weather. Whatever you feel comfortable wearing is all right.

There is one rule though—never, never, never wear anything that will make you sweat. I'm referring here to vapor suits. A long time ago, coaches (men, of course) got the idea that exercising in a rubberized sweat suit would make you lose weight. Well, they're right—but the lost weight is body water. And that is a very dangerous thing. You become hyperthermic (elevated body temperature as in fever) and that can cause heat stroke, which is a failure of your temperature regulating system that can be fatal. Wearing a vapor suit while "working out" is so dangerous that it is forbidden in exercise clubs and by major National sport associations such as the National Collegiate Athletic Association (NCAA). I still see people doing this, however (nearly always men—I think they think this is a macho way to lose weight).

GETTING STARTED

Walking. You've done it all your life. And sometimes, briskly. But this is going to be different. You've always thought of walking as—well, pedestrian, which according to *The Random House Dictionary*, is lacking in vitality or imagination. I suppose that's why so many people try to jog instead, or go to gyms and try "aerobics." They think walking is "ho hum" boring. Well, my dears, we're going to change that thinking. Walking is not only fun, but walking is interesting, and there is a special technique to it. So, listen up, because "brisk walking, power walking, dynamic walking, striding"—whatever you want to call it—is dif-fer-ent!

The Technique of Brisk Walking

First of all, your posture is very important. Let's check yours. Examine your reflection from the side in a full length mirror or window. Imagine there is a string dropping from above the top of your head, through your ear, through your shoulder, hip and knee joints, and down to your ankle. Elongate your back very slightly tucking your pelvis under you without tightening your shoulders. Your chest is up (but not in a stiff military way) and your tummy is in. You're "lookin' good." Check again, are your shoulders down? Be sure your knees aren't locked backwards. You should feel that your pelvis fully supports your upper body, but not feel heavy there. In fact, imagine that you are suspended from the string above your head so that your feet just barely rest on the ground as if you were hanging from that string. This is an important feeling that I will come back to again later.

OK, now begin to walk—not very fast yet—breathing normally, and letting your arms swing naturally, hands relaxed (not clenched). Notice any stiffness in your body. Walk for a few minutes and come back to the mirror or window. (Don't worry, you won't have to do this every time you walk.)

Check your posture again. Did you sag? Or were you so conscious of your posture that you tightened up your shoulders and got stiff? Go through the posture check again. Look for the imaginary string. This (the posture check) is important because most of us are very sloppy about our posture. We allow our chests to fall in, our bellies to collapse forward, we arch our backs too much, and our shoulders are either too far back or too far forward. Do you know what happens? We get back aches—and wonder why, and lose a lot of muscle tone. It is our muscle tone that makes us look good, so it is obviously very important. The form of walking described here will help you build good posture, good muscle tone, and you will really look good doing it.

Alright, begin walking again. This time pay attention to your feet. Notice your heel striking the ground, your foot flexing as you roll your weight forward onto it, and the push-off from the ball of your foot and toes. Be sure your feet are moving in parallel lines, not swinging outward and around. Notice whether your foot rolls inward (pronation) or outward (supination) as it lands on the ground and your weight comes forward onto it. If it is excessive either way, you may need arch supports in your shoes, or an orthotic device. If any sort of foot pain develops make a point of seeing a podiatrist to check this out. (It is beyond the scope of this book to describe the dynamics of the foot—see a specialist if you develop an overuse injury before it becomes a real problem. Most foot problems are very easily solved but require an expert to really know what the underlying cause is. Feet are very complicated structures.) Obviously, your right side should mirror your left side. Observe if this is really the case.

Let's now pay attention to your arms, before going back to leg action once again. I've already pointed out the obvious—your arms move in opposition to your legs (left leg forward, right arm forward, etc).

Your arm movements should be *purposeful* movements—not limp, uncontrolled swinging motions—and not stiff, awkward movements. There should be a slight bend—about 10 degrees is enough—at the elbows (just be sure you don't lock your elbow joints), and your thumbs should be directed straight ahead leading the rest of your hand. Your palms should face the side of each leg and be relaxed, not clenched. Use the muscles in the front of your arm and shoulder, and those in the back of your arm and shoulder, to do the swinging motions. You are not simply letting gravity carry your arms through. The movement is not forceful, but it is purposeful. I suppose that's a subtle difference, but it is an important one. You are not lazily "throwing" your arms forward, nor are you "forcing" them forward as in a military "goose-step." Figure 7.2 provides a good view of the arm and leg movements I am describing.

Pay attention to the path your hands take on your arm swing. They should be moving in a fairly straight line parallelling the movements of your feet, not swinging in an arc around your body. Your right hand should

FIGURE 7.2
The technique of brisk walking.

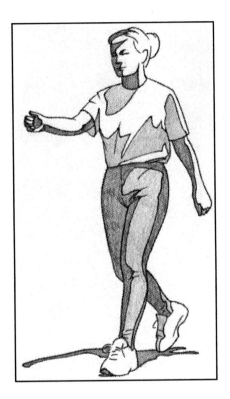

come to about breast height in front of your right shoulder. Your left hand should come to breast height in front of its corresponding shoulder. You'll see many people walking with a rotating arm swing. That is not correct.

With very fast walking, you will want to bend your arms more at the elbows, and your hands will come more toward the center of your body on the forward swing. They should never, however, overlap in front. This is a little like the race walking arm movement, but not nearly as extreme. Unfortunately, I see lots of people brisk walking using a race walking arm swing. It's really a little ridiculous. For one thing, it isn't at all necessary because it is not contributing to walking at a very fast pace which is the purpose of the race walking arm swing, and for another, it defeats the purpose intended—which is usually to burn calories. These people (who are not race walking) end up "carrying" their arms. Their arm movement is not purposeful—it is limp, requiring little or no muscular effort, and therefore, contributes very little (if anything at all) to the caloric expenditure of walking. Don't use the pumping, bent elbow arm swing unless you are actually race walking (which is not what I am describing here).

Now let's get back to your leg action once again with something a little new, ready? When you've mastered everything above, add this: Make your strides long and smooth. Just as you make heel contact with the ground and begin to shift your weight from the rear leg to the new forward leg, contract the quadriceps muscle (the large muscle on the front of your thigh) on your new supporting leg, and "*pull*" yourself forward. There's no way this can be shown in a "figure"—you'll simply have to "feel" it. It will add a little surge and lift to your walk. Try it. As your heel touches the ground, contract the "quad" and *pull*. The sensation you get is of being "pulled forward" by the front leg, not a bounce or spring from the rear (push-off) leg. It's tricky to describe, but not hard to do once you have the concept.

Remember—and the leg effort just described will help this—stand tall by lifting tall out of your hips as if suspended from that string above your head. Imagine lifting your head into a crown. Instead of pounding the ground, you are floating, almost dancing, above it. It's a wonderful feeling. If you don't get it at first, simply reread this complete description periodically, and it will suddenly come to you.

You are ready to get serious about daily brisk walking.

Warm-Up—Before Each Walk

Begin thinking like an athlete—even if you think you are far from being an athlete. It's the frame of mind you want to capture. And, athletes always warm-up. Now don't let me scare you—this is really easy. Unfortunately, many people, athletes included, think prolonged complicated warm-ups are necessary, and they are not. There are two parts of a warm-up. The first part is to stretch the muscles that will be used during brisk walking, and the second is to begin increasing the circulation of blood to those muscles. Your warm-up will last about two minutes—that's right, the 2-Minute Warm-Up.

And here it is, the 2-Minute Warm-Up for Brisk Walking:

- ❤ SWING ARMS. Gently swing your arms forward and back and side-to-side several times each.
- ❤ SHOULDER SHRUG/HEAD TURN. Shrug your shoulders a couple of times, and rotate your head to the left and then to the right several times.
- ❤ BACK ROLL. Beginning with feet flat on the ground, about shoulder width apart, place your hands on your thighs. Bend your knees very slightly, and then S-L-O-W-L-Y, slide your hands down your thighs to your knees by rolling your spine forward beginning at your neck, then your upper back, and then your lower

back while you suck in your tummy. Hold a couple of seconds, then straighten up s-l-o-w-l-y. Repeat twice. NOTE: Knees, not toes, and don't lock your knees backward.

♥ LEG STRETCH. With both feet pointing straight ahead, step forward on your right foot, keeping both feet flat on the ground. Place your hands on your hips—or hold onto a chair or wall for balance. Continuing to keep both feet flat on the ground, bend your knees and lower your body several inches keeping your weight evenly divided on both legs. Hold 5 to 8 seconds. Don't bounce. You will feel a stretch in the calf of your rear leg, and a little in the front thigh of your front leg. Reverse legs, and repeat once each leg.

♥ CARDIO WARM-UP. Begin to walk...very slowly at first, gradually picking up your pace. Take about 1 minute to get to your brisk walking pace. This gradually increases blood flow to your walking muscles.

That's all you need to do for a warm-up. If you want to do more, if you feel that you should do more, you certainly may, but you don't need to do more. I've given each exercise a name so that you can easily remember them. Practice each now.

Cool-Down—After Brisk Walking

I can't emphasize enough how important a Cool-Down after exercise is. A Cool-Down prevents stiffness, prevents overuse injuries, and helps you recover much faster. There are two parts to a Cool-Down just as there are to the warm-up, but in reverse order. First there is the cardio cool-down, and then stretching.

Cardio Cool-Down. Slow your walk to your Warm-Up pace, and maintain this for at least 3 minutes. The purpose of the Cardio Cool-Down is to begin to lower your body temperature after exercise and to gradually allow your cardiovascular system to return to its pre-walking state. Exerting yourself and then abruptly stopping can be very dangerous because it is a "shock" to your heart. It is very important that you not skip the Cardio Cool-Down.

The second part of your Cool-Down is similar to your Warm-Up, only now your muscles are quite warm from the exercise you have done, and stretching is particularly effective. Years of research indicates that stretching is most effective when muscles are warm and supple following exercise. Three stretches are essential for walkers.

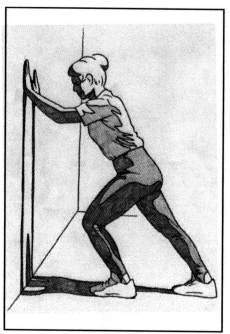

Figure 7.3
Calf Stretcher

Calf Stretcher. Place both hands against a wall or tree, with one foot well behind you. Check that both feet point straight ahead toward the wall or tree. Keeping your rear leg straight and your heel on the ground, lean in toward the wall or tree. Keep your back straight. Do not bounce. You will feel a stretch along the back of your rear lower leg. This stretches your Achilles tendon and gastrocnemius muscle (the big muscle in the back of your calf). It should feel tight, but it should not hurt. Hold for 20 seconds. Reverse legs. Repeat.

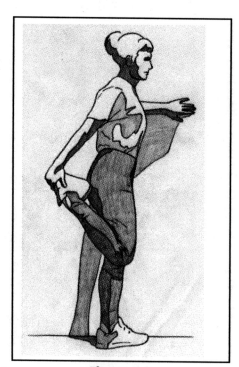

Figure 7.4
Quad Stretcher

Quad Stretcher. Stand erect while supporting yourself with your left arm against a wall or tree. With your right arm, reach behind you and grasp the ankle of your right leg. Gently and slowly pull it up toward your buttocks until you feel tension along the front of your thigh—your quadriceps muscle. Your knee should be pointing toward the ground. Be sure you don't lean forward at the waist, it is important to maintain a fully upright posture. Hold for 20 seconds. Reverse legs.

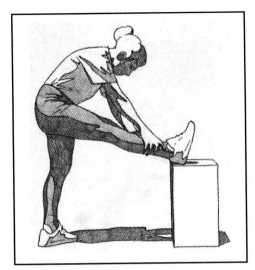

**Figure 7.5
Hamstring Stretcher**

a) standing

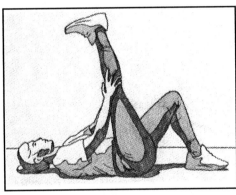

b) lying

Hamstring Stretcher. There are several ways to do this stretch. Usually the most convenient way is to stand on one leg and prop the other leg on a step or bench. Slide both hands down your leg toward your propped-up ankle as far as they'll go. Hold for 20 seconds. You will feel a stretch along the back of your thigh (your hamstrings). Do not bounce. Reverse legs.

A better way is to lay on your back with both legs bent to 90 degrees and feet flat on the floor. Bring one leg to your chest, and place your hands behind your knee. Gradually straighten your leg pushing your heel toward the ceiling or sky (that's important, don't point your toe, point your heel). Gently pull your leg toward your chest and hold for 20 seconds. You will feel a stretch in the muscles in the back of your thigh. Reverse legs. Repeat.

You shouldn't rush your Cool-Down, so I don't want to give a time period that you will follow to the second—but it should take at least 7 or 8 minutes. If you feel like you need more Cool-Down, by all means, do more.

DOING IT—WALKING FOR YOUR HEART

You're ready to go—you have good, well-fitting walking shoes, and you've decided what to wear. We've discussed the technique of walking, and you have tried it out and it feels fine. You've also practiced the Warm-Up and Cool-Down exercises. What do you do now?

First, make a copy of the RPE scale (p. 100) on a small piece of paper or card you can carry with you a few times. Actually, all you really need to copy are the three descriptors and RPE numbers that you will eventually memorize:

Always warm-up before and cooldown after each brisk walk.

> Fairly light = 11
> Somewhat hard = 13
> Hard = 15

Then, after doing your Warm-Up—the 2-Minute Warm-Up for brisk walking—walk for about 15 minutes at a pace that is comfortable for you but is slightly above your usual walking pace. This is an exploratory walk— you have yet to establish your moderate intensity brisk walking pace.

After about 10 minutes, look at the RPE scale and descriptors on your card. If you "feel" that the walking pace is "Fairly light" or 11 on the RPE scale, then speed up your pace a little. If you feel that the walking pace is "hard" or 15 on the RPE scale, then slow down a little bit. Experiment with your pace. Find the pace that is between 13 and 14 (somewhat hard). Obviously, this walking session must be done alone because you are attempting to concentrate on pace (as well as technique) and trying to find the pace that is exactly right for you, and not anyone else. When you have found this pace—walk for about 10 or 15 minutes more. You should feel like your heart rate is elevated—but not racing, you are warm and sweating a little (this, of course, is also a function of climate), and that you are glowing—you are well and energetic.

Then Cool-Down. You have completed your first Brisk Walk. You are on your way to establishing a Heart Healthy lifestyle.

On day 2, begin with your Warm-Up. Then walk at the pace you determined yesterday...taking the first 5 minutes or so to find the pace that corresponds to the RPE rating of 13 or 14. If you had no residual fatigue from your Exploratory Walk, then walk for about 30 minutes at that pace. Then Cool-Down. If you do have some residual fatigue from your Exploratory Walk, then match your time (duration) rather than exceed it.

YOU'VE DONE IT!! IT'S REALLY THAT EASY!!

If you have been completely inactive for a long time, if your doctor has told you you have heart or vascular disease, or if you have had a previous heart attack, then you may need to ease into the full 30-minute Brisk Walk more gradually. Whatever works best for you is the thing to do. If you walk 10 minutes on day 1, and 12 minutes on day 2, and 15 minutes on day 3—then, that's great. This should be fun and healthful for you. The object is not to cause undue fatigue. Ease into the "at least 30 minutes most days of the week" as you need to. Just don't put it off.

Establish Several Walking Courses

If you are interested in doing so, measure several different routes—for variation. Variety is the spice of life so why walk the same route every day. You can use your car odometer for this, or the rule of ten city blocks to a mile. Two miles per course is a good start.

Then you can record your time to cover these courses. Start by timing how long it takes you to walk one mile comfortably on flat ground. Most likely it will be between 15 and 20 minutes, but don't worry if you are slower than this. The important thing is to maintain a steady pace at the Perceived Exertion Rating prescribed—13 to 14. Whatever your time for the distance, you can build from there. That's the whole point of recording your distance and time. (see below)

Keeping It Up

It is a good idea to schedule your walks in advance, and then to keep the appointment. Be sure to plan time for your 2-Minute Warm-Up and the Cool-Down.

To make Brisk Walking a real Heart Healthy habit takes willpower—and often strategy. It is often a good idea to schedule your walks in the morning before other commitments crop up to distract you. Another good idea is to schedule your walks with a friend—it is harder to "not show up" when there is someone waiting for you. A "walking buddy" helps keep you on schedule and can be loads of fun. The only problem with walking with a "buddy" is that you need to walk at your pace, not your buddy's pace. You could also get a dog or walk a friend's dog—it should be well trained though and not stop at every tree, fence post, or fire hydrant.

Another good strategy is to keep a walking record. This not only serves as a reminder, but acts a little like an appointment book. Here's a sample form. Feel free to make up your own form.

Week of (date)	Warm-Up	Cool-Down	Walking Time	Distance (optional)	Comments
Day 1					
Day 2					
Day 3					
Day 4					
Day 5					
Day 6					
Day 7					

Indoor Walking

Many communities today have established indoor walking areas or walkways. These can be used in bad weather or to avoid busy city streets. Indoor walking allows you to remain dry, warm, and safe. I used to live in Phoenix where it is very hot in the summer. Lots of people walked for exercise in the indoor shopping malls. To find out about indoor walking contact the following:

- ❤ Shopping Mall Managers Office: If there is no specified "walking trail," suggest they establish one. Inquire when the doors open or when the best hours may be for walking.
- ❤ Senior Citizen Centers: Even if you are not a senior citizen, these centers are often good sources of information.
- ❤ Department Store Managers: Some cities have enclosed walkways between blocks (and stores) that can be used for walking.
- ❤ National Organization of Mall Walkers (yes, really!): PO Box 191, Hermann, MO 65041.
- ❤ Hospitals or Wellness Centers: A hospital based wellness clinic or health center may sponsor an indoor walking program. Use your phone book to make inquiries.
- ❤ Universities and colleges: There are often wellness or fitness centers that sponsor walking programs on campus, often in a gym or recreation center. Inquire of the Health or Fitness Center, the Physical Education Department, or the Recreation Department.
- ❤ Your local YMCA, YWCA, or YMHA.

Using Exercise Machines

Another way to walk indoors is to walk on a treadmill at a fitness center or health spa. Treadmill walking is a popular choice of many people. There are many advantages to walking on a treadmill. It is safe—no cars, no exhaust fumes, no dogs to chase you, no wind or rain or sleet or snow, no ice to slip on. Many treadmills have "programming features" that allow you to challenge yourself by altering your speed and grade (the hills you climb). Some even have built in heart rate monitors. And, this makes them fun—at least for a while.

There are disadvantages too. Unfortunately, after a while treadmill walking can be very boring—but I have some solutions for that, see the section below called Relieving the Boredom.... If you treadmill walk at a health or fitness club you have to pay—unless you are very lucky, it's not free. There is usually an initiation fee plus monthly "dues." Buying your own treadmill can be quite costly—expect to pay between $1000 and $2000—and they take up quite a bit of space. Most become expensive clothes-hangers. In addition, treadmills can be quite noisy, and you miss the marvelous (and healthful) experience of being outdoors. Nonetheless, you might like to try it. (You'll note that I'm pretty biased toward outdoor exercise.)

You can obtain more information about owning your own treadmill by calling the manufacturers listed in RESOURCES under Treadmill Manufactures.

Another alternative is a cross-country ski machine. The primary advantage is that you get to exercise your arms rather vigorously along with your legs. The primary disadvantage is that it takes some skill to be very good at this. If you enjoy cross-country skiing on snow, you'll probably enjoy giving this a try. Many health clubs have cross-country ski machines as well as treadmills. If you want to exercise at home, be sure to try one out before buying one, however, it's a far cry from enjoying the fresh air and snow of the great out-of-doors. Two companies that make good cross-country ski machines are listed in RESOURCES under Cross-Country Ski Machine Manufacturers).

Other alternative exercise machines that I recommend (at least as far as I recommend exercise machines at all) include stair steppers/climbers, elliptical striding systems, and stationary cycles. These are low impact alternatives to jogging or running. Using a stepper is like walking up a staircase treadmill. A few machines add a climbing element—like a ladder treadmill—you step up with your feet, and you pull up with your arms. In elliptical striding, your feet never leave foot-pads that you move in oblong circles. Sounds weird, but it's really very smooth. You can get quite a work-out on these machines—but you need to ask yourself—do I really want to do 30 minutes of this every day? Be sure to try out these machines at your health club before you buy one for the convenience of exercising at home. Otherwise, you may end up with a very expensive clothes hanger. (See RESOURCES under Stair-stepper Manufacturers and Stair-climber Manu-facturers.)

Another low-impact exercise machine is a stationary cycle. These are good for people with leg or foot problems, arthritis, people who are over-weight, and possibly, for some people with back problems (but not all). Some machines have push-pull or cycling arm pedals as well as leg pedals. Most health and fitness clubs will have stationary cycles—although not always the latest kind. Stationary cycles are a lot cheaper to buy than treadmills or stair steppers. See RESOURCES under Stationary Cycle Manu-facturers.

I've already indicated my bias against exercise machines, but they are excellent choices for many people. If you join a health or fitness club, you may find that you enjoy walking on a treadmill one day, stationary cycling the next day, stairclimbing the third day, and maybe swimming the fourth day, etc. Or, you may find that some form of exercise machine is a great choice on days when the weather is bad and you prefer to stay indoors.

Because there is no air moving around you as you walk or cycle or ski or climb on a stationary machine, you will feel very hot. You will think that you are sweating a lot more than when you exercise outdoors. This is not really true, it's just that your sweat is not evaporating like it does when you are outdoors. This extra build-up of body heat will be reflected in your perceived exertion rating. For example: If your usual outdoor walking pace at a perceived exertion rating of 13 (somewhat hard) is 3.5 mph, when you walk indoors on a treadmill at that same pace, your perceived exer-tion rating may be 15 (hard), and no, you're not crazy...it's the lack of air movement around your body preventing the loss of body heat that is mak-ing the same exercise seem harder to do. There are two things you can do. One is to find a high speed fan and direct it on your body. This will mimic the outdoor air flow around you. The other is to adjust your walking speed. The wonderful thing about the use of perceived exertion rating (as I ex-plained before) is that it is a very reliable indication of the stain on your body.

Relieving the Boredom of Exercise Machines

If you choose to use exercise machines, here are some ideas about how to relieve the boredom:

Make your treadmill walks (or other forms of exercise) a cultural experience: Get a "walkman" type "stick it in your ear" tape or CD player that will attach to your arm or waist. Start with your favorite music. Acquaint yourself with other types of music—classical, jazz, folk, bluegrass, rock'n roll. To try out new kinds of music see if you can borrow tapes from the library.

Audio books are great for exercising on a machine! For example, try James Michener's *Chesapeake* or *Alaska*. Those will keep you busy for a while! *Dances with Wolves* by Michael Blake is excellent too. Try murder, mystery, science fiction, adventure, religion—anything you want. Many book stores, video stores, and libraries now have audio books. Or, write to Random House Audiobooks, Recorded Books, or Books on Tape. (See RESOURCES under Audio Books for use during walking). Some companies are now renting tapes in mail-back boxes.

Time on an exercise machine can be used for self-improvement. Tapes are available on motivation, concentration, loving yourself, selling techniques, memory improvement, foreign languages, etc. Do not use self-hypnosis tapes while exercising. There are dangers to having a microphone in your ears while walking out-of-doors, and so I do not recommend using headphones when you are outside. The first reason is a matter of safety. People have been known to literally forget where they are and walk right into cars. Remember to LOOK at cross streets, and LISTEN for surrounding traffic (maybe dogs, too). Don't become so unaware of your surroundings that you endanger yourself. It's important to BE ALERT while walking. There are some dangers out there.

The second danger is that you may forget where you are and get lost. A 40-minute walk could easily turn into an hour and a half.

MAKE WALKING FUN

Walking is fun. You can enjoy nature—the woods, streams, birds, and country roads—or the urban landscape. You can escape from the house, the dishes, the children, your in-laws, your spouse.

Walking can be solitary. Walking can be social. Walking can be anything you want it to be.

A way to turn outdoor walking into a cultural experience is to go on walking tours—many cities have historical routes, tours of city gardens or arboretums, urban architecture walks, and city sculpture tours. Explore your city. This is also a good way to get your walking in when on a business trip or vacation. For information inquire at your hotel, contact the Chamber of Commerce, or contact the American Institute of Architects (listed in RESOURCES under Walking.)

Making Brisk Walking a Social Experience

I've already mentioned walking with a "walking buddy." This helps you adhere to your walking program because now you have a responsibility—to meet your buddy. Whenever someone else is involved you have "to schedule" your walks.

Another way to make walking a social experience is to get involved with walking clubs. You will be surprised at the breadth of clubs and organizations available. See RESOURCES under Walking for names and addresses to contact about a chapter near you. Also call your YWCA, YMCA, or YMHA.

HIKING is, of course, walking—an absolutely wonderful way to walk. There are several major hiking organizations that may have a local affiliate club in your region. (See RESOURCES under Hiking.)

ORIENTEERING is a form of competitive walking in which you find your way around a course with a map and compass. Some people run, but not everyone does this at top speed. Contact the US Orienteering Federation (see RESOURCES under Walking) to find a local club.

OTHER THINGS YOU SHOULD KNOW

How to Care for Your Walking Feet

If you get sore feet or blisters, you won't want to continuing walking, so good foot care is important. Feet are complicated structures with many tiny muscles, ligaments and tendons. Good shoes, and good foot care will avoid potential problems. Preventive foot care is the best foot care. Keep your feet dry (use socks that wick moisture), give them lots of air between walks to prevent the growth of bacteria, and keep your nails well trimmed. If you have any sort of foot problem that is persistent, see a podiatrist or orthopedist.

How to Care for Your Walking Shoes

Using your walking shoes only for walking will not only save wear, but will allow them to air out thoroughly. If you put your shoes on early in the morning, do your brisk walking, and not take your shoes off until much later in the day, moisture will be retained not only next to your skin (bad for your feet), but within the shoe (bad for the shoe). And you know what that means. Phew-ee !! I recommend that you remove the insoles for complete airing and drying at least once per week.

If your shoes get wet and dirty in the rain or dew (don't skip inclement days), first wipe off the excess dirt, then stuff them lightly with absorbent paper towels so that they will not lose their shape as they dry out. Place them in a warm, but not hot, place to dry out. And never dry your shoes in the dryer or place them in the sun. To wash them, take an old nail brush and scrub them in a pail of warm soapy water, drain them as best you can, stuff lightly with absorbent paper, and place them in a warm spot to dry. You will probably need to remove the wet paper and re-stuff them with dry paper a couple of times. Believe me, this works. If you place athletic shoes in a dryer they will get too hot, the material will crack (maybe not the first time, but certainly with repeated washing), and they will curl up. Result? Short shoe life—and tight shoes.

Drinking Fluids

Your body has several ways to eliminate the metabolic heat you generate when you exercise. The most effective way is by sweating. However, if you become dehydrated because you do not replace the body fluids you lose, then you are endangering yourself. Dehydration is particularly stressful to your cardiovascular system, so becoming low in body fluids will defeat much of what you want to accomplish by brisk walking.

You've probably seen exercisers—walking, joggers, runners, cyclists—with water bottles, or Camelbaks™ (tiny backpacks for carrying a water bladder with a tube that comes over your shoulder and attaches very close to your mouth). It's a very good idea, and I highly recommend you always carry water with you on your daily walks.

Signs of dehydration include nausea, flushed skin, feeling light-headed, being unable to concentrate. Other signs include having dark yellow urine or not being able to urinate at all (pretty advanced dehydration by that time). Muscle cramps can be brought on by dehydration, but there are other causes as well.

How much water should you drink? Ideally, you should drink as much water as you lose—but that is pretty hard to assess while you are walking. You can tell how much water you've lost by weighing yourself before your walk and again after your walk and subtracting the difference. That's lost water weight. This tells you how much you should have drunk during the walk, and of course, how much water to drink for a full recovery. But you need a guide to know how much water to drink *while* you are brisk walking—and it is impossible to be exact. A good guide is provided by the American College of Sports Medicine.

BEFORE your brisk walk. Drink about 2 cups (16 oz) of fluid approximately two hours before you begin your walk. This is sometimes called pre-hydration.

DURING your brisk walk. Drink 20 to 40 oz per hour of a cool, palatable, non-carbonated fluid. This translates to about 5 to 10 oz of fluid every 15 to 20 minutes. Drinking while walking is really quite easy. A cycling water bottle makes it even easier, as do the Camelbak's I mentioned earlier.

AFTER your brisk walk. Drink at least 2 cups (16 oz) for every one pound of body weight you lose during the activity.

The next major question—and this is complicated—is WHAT should you drink? Is water sufficient?

Your body utilizes glucose and muscle glycogen—forms of internal carbohydrate—for energy (calories) during exercise. As you lose water from sweating, electrolytes are also lost. Electrolytes (ions) are the major minerals in your blood—sodium, potassium and chloride. If you exercise for more than an hour at a time and/or sweat very heavily (as is common in very hot or humid weather), then you need to replace some of your body's glucose and electrolytes. Otherwise, water is probably sufficient. The rule is something like this:

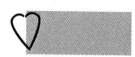

Always carry water with you and sip it frequently as you walk.

- ❤ Short period of exercise—replace body water
- ❤ Long endurance exercise—replace body water plus internal energy sources (calories) and electrolytes

So my rule-of-thumb advice to you is as follows:

If you exercise for up to or less than 60 minutes at a time carry water with you and sip frequently. Consume at least one cycling water bottle—20 oz—of water.

If you exercise for more than 60 minutes at a time, or exercise in a very hot-dry (like Phoenix) or hot-humid (like Atlanta) climate, consume a sport drink such as Gatorade, Exceed, Powerade, or Allsport. These drinks provide water, glucose and electrolytes. Remember, these "energy drinks" contain calories, so if one of your goals is to lose weight, you will have to account for this in order to sustain weight loss.

What About Bad Weather?

Remember the goal? It hasn't been stated in many pages now. TO WALK BRISKLY AT LEAST 30 MINUTES MOST DAYS OF THE WEEK. And, most days of the week, clearly means PREFERABLY ALL days of the week. That means—you don't get rainy or snowy or foggy or cloudy or dreary days off. There are many alternatives. One is "aerobic-dancing"—as described earlier in this chapter. Create a little space—move some furniture if you have to, put on a good tape or CD, draw the curtains if you feel like it, and do it. Have fun!!!

Another alternative is to go to a gym and use the exercise machines. Or, walk anyway. I advocate walking in the rain—maybe not real downpours, but light showers, certainly. Don't be afraid of walking in a little rain. If you do, you'll probably discover that you really don't want to dress too warmly. Personally, I don't mind getting wet—I just don't want to get cold. So spring, summer and fall rain is fine. I seldom wear a rain jacket unless it is a jacket that "breathes" or I get wetter on the inside than I do on the outside. This is hard to describe, but once you experience it, you'll know what I mean.

If you don't want to brisk walk in the rain or snow, then you will need to find an alternative and there are quite a few acceptable alternatives...remember, commit yourself and DO IT.

What If You Aren't Feeling Well?

This has been a topic of discussion among athletes and coaches for some time. It turns out that exercise does not harm you if you have a cold, but it is *not* a good idea if you have a fever. Personally, when I have a "common cold," I drink some hot herbal tea, take some vitamin C, some Echinacea and a zinc lozenge if I have a sore throat, and go for a brisk walk. I always feel better. If the weather is terrible, I "aerobic-dance" in my living room. If I have a fever, I go to bed. Anyone with a fever belongs in bed.

What If You Experience Chest Pain or Feel Faint?

If you have chest pain, palpitations, or you feel faint or lightheaded during or immediately after exercise, you should stop what you are doing, drink a little fluid—water is best, and sit down. Do not lie down—at least not immediately—because that often puts considerable pressure on your heart from all the blood returned to it from your lower body.

If you are alone, call a friend.

If you are at a health club, let someone know—either the instructor, or someone at the desk. Do *not* go home immediately or go into the locker room by yourself. You will most likely be just fine, but there is no sense complicating a possibly dangerous situation by going off and being alone. Sit out the rest of the class in the back.

If you are out on a brisk walk, go into a store and sit down. Tell someone you are not feeling well, and stay with people.

If your symptoms persist for more than 5 minutes after you have stopped exercise call or have someone call 9-1-1 for you. Better to be absolutely safe than sorry later.

MAKING PHYSICAL ACTIVITY A REAL PART OF YOUR LIFE

When you exercise on a daily basis, you will feel better than you ever did before. It is time to consciously make physical activity a real part of your life—a part of your lifestyle. There are so many ways to do this in addition to the periods of time you set aside specifically for your Heart Healthy brisk walking. Here are a few ways to incorporate more physical activity into your life as you go about your regular work, home, childcare, food preparation, and personal care activities:

❤ park a few blocks away from your destination and walk
❤ use the stairs instead of the elevator or escalator
❤ carry your groceries to the car rather than use a cart
❤ take a 5 minute walk as a work break
❤ walk the golf course and carry your clubs rather than use a cart
❤ play with the dog (cat?)
❤ do the exercises described in this book during TV commercials (and, of course, don't eat)
❤ do your own interoffice deliveries
❤ get off the bus or subway one stop too soon and walk the rest of the way to work

CONGRATULATIONS. You should feel proud of yourself for making the commitment to walk briskly for your heart.

CHAPTER 8

Eating for Your Heart

Confused about what you should and shouldn't eat? Most people are. So much has been written about diet and heart disease it is no wonder you are confused. To make matters worse, some of the earlier information provided by physicians and government agencies hasn't really stood the test of time. Madison Avenue hasn't helped much either—they often fool the American public by advertising foods that never had cholesterol in the first place—as cholesterol-free. And the "fat free," "low fat," "reduced fat," "97% fat free" ads are totally confusing. I'll unscramble all that later in this chapter.

The American diet is notoriously high in fat, protein, sugar, salt—and calories. These nutrients are necessary for us to eat—we need fat, protein, sugar and salt to survive, and obviously, we need calories—but we greatly abuse these nutritional needs. For example, according to Jane Brody, author of *Jane Brody's Good Food Book*, a typical American dinner contains:

- ❤ a generous portion of animal protein—perhaps as much as 8 ounces of red meat, a quarter chicken, or ½ pound of fish (the latter two probably fried)
- ❤ potatoes that are deep-fried and salted, or baked and topped with butter and sour cream and salt
- ❤ buttered or creamed vegetables, also salted
- ❤ a salad covered with a salty, oil-based dressing and
- ❤ a sugary soft drink or iced-tea (which is much better) loaded with sugar (which is not), and
- ❤ ice cream, cake or pie (likely with ice cream on top).

I'm sure you'll agree that's a pretty rich but not uncommon meal, and obviously high in calories, fat, protein, and salt. In fact, according to Brody, the amount of protein is triple that needed in a single meal; the fat content is half the total calories—which means this meal is 50% fat; the salt content meets the recommended amount for a whole day; and the sugar content (although less obvious) is quite high—possibly as much as 27 teaspoons of refined sugar. The caloric content is probably more than many people of the world—healthy people, not starving people from Third World nations—consume in several days. No wonder Americans have so much heart disease, diabetes, hypertension, and obesity!

Maybe we don't eat like that every day, but the fact remains we consume more steak, hamburgers, hot dogs, fried chicken, ice cream, soda pop, potato chips, and salty tortilla chips—than any other nation in the world. And to make matters worse, we consume fewer fruits and vegetables per capita than people in almost any other nation.

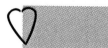

Americans consume more fat, protein, sugar, salt and total calories than most other people in the world. No wonder we have such high rates of heart disease, diabetes, hypertension and obesity.

Well, the usual approach is to emphasize all the things we do wrong—and that's exactly what I've done so far, right? But you probably already know these things, so from here on out—the approach will be positive. Although I can't get totally away from "what's wrong with the American diet" I will be emphasizing the things you should do rather than the things you shouldn't do.

The first of two basic principles is:

EAT MORE HEART HEALTHY FOODS

The following pages will clarify exactly what these foods are, why they are protective to your heart and blood vessels, what to look for in the grocery, and how to prepare them in a heart healthy manner. Some very simple to follow and realistic "resolutions" will be given. These will be your daily and weekly goals—like New Year's Resolutions—only more precise.

The second of our two basic principles is:

EAT LESS HEART DAMAGING FOODS

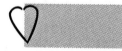

It's really simple. To lower your risk of heart disease and stroke, eat more Heart Healthy foods and eat less heart damaging foods.

While that might sound "negative" and that I am contradicting what I said just above, the approach will be positive. As with the first principle, I will clarify what these foods are and why you shouldn't be consuming them in large quantities. Because so many of us are dependent on some of these foods, tasty, and easy to prepare heart healthy substitutions will be emphasized. What could be more positive? This will not be drudgery. While it may be challenging—because you may need to change and change is always challenging—it will also be simple, fun, realistic, and adventurous. Ready to proceed?

To begin, you must develop an increased awareness of foods that includes an increased awareness of what you eat and a basic understanding about "food groups." But don't worry, you won't need to memorize anything.

INCREASING YOUR AWARENESS OF FOODS

Many people say that Americans are already "aware" of food. Studies show that about 48% of us are on a "diet" at some point during a year. But that's not what I mean by food awareness. Worrying about how much and what kind of food you are eating is not "food awareness," it is "worrying" about not eating right, about violating your d-i-e-t. Awareness requires understanding, recognition and consciousness, not worry. I am speaking here of increased food "mindfulness."

First of all, I consider D-I-E-T a four-letter word. We've learned over the years that "dieting" to lose weight simply doesn't work. Although you may initially lose weight, in the long run dieting only sets you up for failure. I am not advocating that you "go on a diet." In fact, I initially tried to write this chapter without even using the word d-i-e-t, but I could not. So let me make my intended meaning quite clear. When I use the word "diet" I mean literally "what a person usually eats or drinks" (*Webster's New World Dictionary*). I am referring to your "way of life" relative to what you eat—your eating lifestyle—and NOT to a special "diet" that you go on to improve your heart health. I am speaking about the way of eating that you select to improve your heart health. It may seem like a subtle difference, but I believe it is a very important difference. This book advocates that you adopt a "way of eating" that is healthful to your heart and blood vessels. To do that, you need to develop food awareness. The best way to achieve this is to have a basic understanding of food groups. Let's use the USDA Food Pyramid as a model.

A basic understanding of the food groups will increase your awareness—your mindfulness—of foods.

FIGURE 8.1
The Food Pyramid

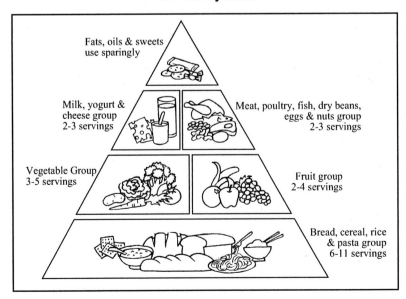

Fats, oils & sweets
use sparingly

Milk, yogurt &
cheese group
2-3 servings

Meat, poultry, fish, dry beans,
eggs & nuts group
2-3 servings

Vegetable Group
3-5 servings

Fruit group
2-4 servings

Bread, cereal, rice
& pasta group
6-11 servings

US Dept of Agriculture and US Dept of Health and Human Services, 1995

THE BASIC FOOD GROUPS

As you can see from Figure 8.1—the Food Pyramid—there are 6 basic food groups. Americans are urged to choose most of their foods from the bottom up—that is, 6 to 11 daily servings from grains, 3 to 5 servings from vegetables, 2 to 4 servings from fruits, etc. These are Heart Healthy foods. The idea is to eat sparingly of the nutrients high in fat and sugars at the very top of the pyramid—the heart damaging foods. Starting at the base of the pyramid, we will consider each food group separately. When you have finished reading this section—don't read too fast—you will have absorbed vital information without having to memorize anything. The numbers I present are merely to help you place the different food groups relative to each other. You'll see what I mean as we go along. (Note: the section describing the first food group, The Grains, will be unusually long because I will define and describe basic terms used in the sections that follow.)

The Grains

As you can see from Figure 8.1, the Grains include breads, cereals, pasta, and rice. These foods are high in fiber and complex carbohydrates. They also contain high amounts of essential vitamins and minerals. In addition, foods in the Grain Group are low in calories (about 68 per serving) and contain a small but significant amount of protein (about 2 grams per serving).

What is fiber? You've probably heard about fiber in the ads for laxatives. Fiber is found *only* in plant foods and is the part of the plant that can not be digested by the human body. There are two types of fiber, but most foods that are high in fiber will contain both types. Soluble fiber forms a gel-like material in water. Good examples are oats, legumes, and fruits (not a Grain). Insoluble fiber does not dissolve in water and therefore moves through your digestive system very quickly. Remember "roughage" or "bulk?" Good examples of insoluble fibers are wheat bran, whole-grains, and most cereals. Vegetables and fruits also contain insoluble fibers.

A high-fiber diet reduces your risk for many health problems and conditions. Most important for your heart is that the soluble fiber in your diet binds with digestive acids made from cholesterol, and then escorts these acids away in your stools. The net result is a lowering of blood cholesterol. Increasing the fiber in your diet results in a reduction in total cholesterol, and best of all, a lowering of low-density lipoprotein-cholesterol—the "bad" cholesterol.

A diet high in fiber also benefits your gastrointestinal system. By aiding the rapid passage of digested foods through your gastrointestinal tract ("gut" is an OK term), you avoid constipation and reduce your risk of hemorrhoids (swollen anal blood vessels), diverticulosis (pouches that protrude through weak spots in the colon), and irritable bowel syndrome (muscle spasms in the bowel or stomach walls). Fiber is a natural laxative (Americans spend $600 million on laxatives per year).

A diet high in fiber enables you to more slowly absorb glucose from the foods you eat, protecting you from glucose intolerance and diabetes. In addition, several recent studies (including the DASH study that I'll discuss later) show that a diet high in fiber lowers high blood pressure. Remember, diabetes, glucose intolerance, and hypertension are important risk factors for heart disease and stroke. A diet high in fiber is definitely heart healthy.

What is a complex carbohydrate? There are two kinds of carbohydrates: simple carbohydrates are simple sugars (also called refined sugars) like table sugar, honey, fructose (fruit sugar), and molasses, and complex carbohydrates are structurally more complicated carbohydrates that contain starch, vitamins and minerals. Both represent the basic form of energy in your body—glucose. Simple "carbos" such as candy, sugary cake frosting, and fruit syrups are absorbed very rapidly into your blood from your gut giving you a quick burst of energy. Ever had a "sugar high?" That's the result of hyperglycemia (high blood glucose) from the rapid absorption of simple sugars. Complex carbos, because they are structurally more elaborate, take more time to digest and are absorbed more slowly into your blood. It's sort of like the hare (simple carbos) and the tortoise (complex carbos) again. Complex carbohydrates "stand by" you longer and result in a less erratic blood glucose profile (fewer rapid ups and downs). This gradual release of glucose into your blood is desirable because it does not require that your body release large amounts of insulin that rapidly deplete your blood sugar causing rebound hunger, *hypoglycemia* (low blood glucose) and fatigue.

Complex carbohydrates (sometimes called starch) are easier for your body to process than proteins and fats, and should be your body's primary source of energy. They also contain important vitamins and minerals that I'll say much more about later. The Grains—wheat, rice, oats, rye, etc—are very important sources of complex carbohydrates as are legumes (the dried beans and peas) and vegetables.

In summary, foods in the Grain Group are low in calories, contain a small amount of protein, and are rich in fiber, complex carbohydrates, vitamins and minerals. No wonder they are at the base of the Food Pyramid and that the Dietary Guidelines for Americans call for 6 to 11 servings of grain per day.

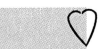

Grains are high in fiber, complex carbohydrates, vitamins and minerals, and low in calories. Brown rice, whole-wheat breads, pasta, couscous, barley, and cooked cereals are examples of these Heart Healthy foods.

What is a grain serving? Very simply, one serving of a grain product is 1 slice of bread, 1 ounce of ready-to-eat cereal, or ½ cup of cooked cereal, rice or pasta. Although easy to accomplish, it takes food awareness to consume 6 to 11 servings of grain a day.

Excellent choices from The Grain Group. Excellent choices from the Grain Group include brown rice, pasta, barley (great in soups and stews), couscous, whole-grain bread, buckwheat pancakes, hot-cooked breakfast cereals like Ralston™, Wheatena™, oatmeal and Cream of Wheat™, and cold ready-to-eat breakfast cereals like Wheaties™, Cherrios™, Shredded Wheat™, and Raisin Bran™.

Foods you should avoid from The Grain Group. Unfortunately, commercially prepared foods that would otherwise be wise grain choices are nearly always "ruined" with the addition of large amounts of simple sugars, salt and "hidden fats." Hidden fats are difficult to detect because they are added to foods in the cooking process and you don't "see" them. Avoid pan-fried and deep-fried foods from the Grain Group.

I do not recommend the following foods from the Grain Group—it is probably easy to see why:

- ❤ Croissants (it is their high fat content that makes them fluffy)
- ❤ Commercially prepared doughnuts, muffins, sweet rolls, waffles or pancakes—too much sugar and fat added. Make your own and you'll know what's in them.
- ❤ Presweetened cereals like Frosted Flakes™, etc.
- ❤ Chow mein noodles—too much added fat and salt
- ❤ Most commercial crackers—too much added fat and salt
- ❤ Egg pasta—high in cholesterol from egg yolks

The Vegetable Group

Moving to the second tier of the Food Pyramid, we find the Vegetable Group and the Fruit Group. The Vegetable Group contains the starchy vegetables such as potatoes, corn, and green peas and the nonstarchy vegetables such as carrots, broccoli, all the greens, and tomatoes. This food group, like the Grains, is high in complex carbohydrates and fiber, in vitamins and minerals, and low in calories (about 28 calories per serving). Contrary to popular thought, vegetables also contain a small, but significant amount of protein (about 2 gm per serving).

The nonstarchy vegetables are most nutritious when eaten raw or only lightly cooked. If you aren't already familiar with steamed vegetables—you need to give this method of preparing nonstarchy vegetables a try because steamed vegetables are delicious, nutritious, and VERY heart healthy. Very little nutrient value is lost as compared, for example, with boiled vegetables.

Some vegetables are particularly noted for their content of the *antioxidants*, vitamin A and beta-carotene (the precursor to vitamin A). Broccoli, carrots, the greens (beet, chard, collard, kale, spinach, turnip), and tomatoes are noted for their vitamin A content. You should eat one serving of one of these vegetables a day.

What is an antioxidant? Antioxidants are substances that prevent the cell damage done by *free radicals*. They do this by destroying free radicals, which are molecules that lack one or more electrons and seek stability by stealing electrons from other molecules found in healthy cells. This stealing of electrons is called oxidation, and results in cell damage that contributes to the aging of a cell. Of special interest relative to heart disease is that antioxidants prevent the oxidation of LDL-C, and thus prevent the cell damage caused by LDL-C in the artery wall, which (as you remember from Chapter 2) is an essential event in the initiation of atherosclerosis. Antioxidants also protect you from cancer, arthritis, cataracts, and other degenerative conditions.

I'm sure you've heard of the antioxidants before. Vitamins A, C and E all have antioxidant capabilities. So does the mineral—selenium. Hence the expression "antioxidant ACES." Many foods in the Vegetable Group contain vitamin A, vitamin C and selenium.

Vegetables, like some fruits and legumes, are also high in *phytochemicals*, substances that protect us from heart disease and cancer.

What is a phytochemical? Researchers have long noted that people who eat a lot of plant foods—vegetables, fruits, grains, and beans—have a strikingly lower risk of heart disease (and cancer). Part of this "protection" stems from the fact that these foods are low in fat and high in vitamins, minerals and fiber. But the overall benefit is greater than the sum of those benefits. Emerging scientific evidence now points to the value of plant chemicals called phytochemicals ("phyto" means plant). There are many such substances, and they are neither vitamins nor minerals.

At least three types of phytochemicals protect us from heart disease. *Plant sterols*—most notably in soy beans—have a cholesterol-lowering effect. They apparently work by inhibiting the absorption of cholesterol in the intestine, and the effect is significant. Mixtures of plant sterols have reduced cholesterol levels by 10%—that's as good as any cholesterol-lowering drug.

Another type of phytochemical is called a *flavonoid*. These compounds are found in vegetables, fruits, nuts and seeds. They also go by the names flavonols, flavones, catechins, and flavonones. Flavonoid intake was inversely related with coronary heart disease in four major world-wide epidemiological studies. That's impressive! These substances inhibit the oxidation of LDL-C, inhibit platelet aggregation, and lower blood cholesterol.

Still another class of phytochemicals important in heart disease are sulfur-containing compounds. These are mostly found in garlic, onions, leeks and chives. They are sometimes called *allyl sulfides*. These compounds lower blood pressure, inhibit platelet aggregation, decrease blood clotting time, and inhibit the synthesis of cholesterol in the liver.

What is a vegetable serving? The _Dietary Guidelines for Americans_ recommend 3 to 5 servings of this Heart Healthy food group. It's really easy to add up Vegetable servings each day because a typical serving is only 1 cup of raw leafy vegetables, ½ cup of most other vegetables—cooked or chopped raw, or ¾ cup of vegetable juice.

Excellent choices from The Vegetable Group. There are so many...steamed or microwaved fresh or frozen broccoli, carrots, green beans, spinach, tomatoes, onions, salad greens, any kind of squash, sweet potatoes, and yams are all exceptionally Heart Healthy foods.

Foods you should avoid from The Vegetable Group. Actually, there are no foods you should avoid from the Vegetable Group, only methods of preparing these foods. Frying vegetables, especially deep-fat frying (as in fried zucchini, a very popular hors d'oeuvre, and onion rings), sure spoils the nutritional value of good foods. And, unfortunately, most commercially prepared vegetables (frozen or canned) add salty and high-fat sauces making these foods quite Heart Unhealthy.

Vegetables are high in complex carbohydrates, fiber, vitamins, minerals, antioxidants, and phytochemicals. They are also low in calories. Any green, yellow, red or orange vegetable is a very Heart Healthy food.

The Fruit Group

Like vegetables, foods in the Fruit Group are high in fiber, rich in vitamins, minerals, antioxidants, and phytochemicals, and low in calories (about 40 calories per serving). Fruits contain only a trace of protein, and both complex and simple carbohydrates. Some fruits contain exceptionally high amounts of vitamin C, and special attention should be made to choose fruits that are high in this nutrient. Vitamin C is not only an antioxidant, but it also promotes the absorption of iron from meats, grains, legumes and vegetables. Daily vitamin C is essential for good health.

You are probably well aware that oranges and orange juice contain a high amount of vitamin C. So does cantaloupe, grapefruit, honeydew melon, strawberries, and watermelon. Notice that the orange and yellow fruits and vegetables contain large amounts of vitamins C and A.

The _Dietary Guidelines for Americans_ recommend that we consume 2 to 4 servings of fruit every day. Unfortunately, there are some Americans who rarely eat fruits.

Fruits are high in fiber, vitamins, minerals, complex carbohydrates, simple carbohydrates, antioxidants and phytochemicals. Any fruit is a Heart Healthy food.

What is a fruit serving? One medium apple, banana, or orange constitute a serving of fruit. So too, does ½ cup of chopped, cooked, or canned fruit, and ¾ cup of fruit juice. So it is very easy to get the recommended amount—it just takes food awareness.

Foods you should avoid From The Fruit Group. Like vegetables, there is no fruit you should avoid—only certain methods of preparation. Avoid commercial fruit pie fillings and commercial fruit whips—too much added sugar. Canned fruit in sugar syrup should also be avoided—obviously for the same reason. Fruits already have simple sugars in them (that's what fructose is—fruit sugar) and there is no need to add more.

The Dairy Group

The third tier of the Food Pyramid is made up of two food groups that provide most of our protein, fat, and cholesterol. The Dairy Group is particularly important—especially for women—because dairy products are excellent sources of the mineral calcium that is essential for bone growth and repair, and the prevention of osteoporosis after menopause. Although some vegetables contain calcium, dairy products contain the most easily absorbed dietary calcium. Although everyone needs calcium, postmenopausal women need 1200 to 1500 milligrams per day to prevent osteoporosis, so milk, cheese and yogurt are very important foods for women.

Dairy products are important sources of protein containing about 8 grams of protein per serving. Although not widely recognized, dairy products are also excellent sources of carbohydrates containing about 12 grams per serving. Unfortunately, diary products also contain *saturated fat* in the form of butterfat (in concentrations that vary from 1 to 80% by weight), and cholesterol. Therefore, it is necessary to make very careful selections from this food group. The *Dietary Guidelines for Americans* recommend that we consume two to three servings from the Dairy Group per day.

What is saturated fat? Dietary "fat" is made up of a class of molecules called fatty acids—long strings of carbon atoms with hydrogen atoms attached. It is the attached hydrogen that identifies the different kinds of fat. A "saturated" fat is thoroughly saturated with hydrogen atoms, which means that every carbon atom has an attached hydrogen and is therefore fully "hydrogenated." These fats are solid at room temperature. An "unsaturated" fat contains less than a full complement of hydrogen atoms meaning that some carbons do not have attached hydrogen atoms. These fats are liquid at room temperature. A *polyunsaturated* fat is an unsaturated fat with several carbon atoms without attached hydrogen. A *monounsaturated fat* is an unsaturated fat with only a single carbon atom without an attached hydrogen.

Not only is a saturated fat hard at room temperature, it is hard on your heart because there is a direct relationship between your consumption of saturated fat and your blood cholesterol and LDL-C levels (the "bad" cholesterol). I'll have more to say about the other dietary fats later (in the Fats & Oils section).

What is a dairy serving? One cup of milk or yogurt makes up one dairy serving. So does 1½ ounces of natural cheese or 2 ounces of processed cheese.

Excellent choices from The Dairy Group. Dairy foods that contain very little or no saturated fat should be your foods of choice from this group. These are the foods based on skim milk. They are high in protein and calcium and low in fat. They are also much lower in cholesterol than the dairy products based on whole milk. Foods based on low fat (1%) milk are also good choices. Cheeses made from skim milk, dry curd cottage cheese, low fat cottage cheese, and reduced-fat cheeses are other good choices.

Yogurt, ice milk, or frozen yogurt are excellent heart healthy foods. Selecting nonfat yogurt, low fat yogurt or low fat fruited yogurt are excellent ways to obtain your essential calcium while consuming minimal levels of saturated fat and cholesterol. I highly recommend that all women consume at least 2 servings of nonfat (skim) or low fat (1% butterfat) milk or yogurt every day.

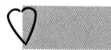

Dairy products are high in protein, calcium, saturated fat, and cholesterol. They are essential to women because of their calcium content, but careful selections are necessary. Skim milk and low fat or nonfat yogurts are heart healthy foods.

Foods you should avoid from The Dairy Group. One cup of whole milk contains 5 grams of saturated fat and 33 milligrams of cholesterol whereas skim milk contains only .3 grams of saturated fat and 4 milligrams of cholesterol. One ounce of cheddar cheese (my favorite, unfortunately) contains 6 grams of saturated fat and 30 milligrams of cholesterol whereas reduced-fat cheddar cheese contains 3 grams of saturated fat and 15 milligrams of cholesterol. Two tablespoons of sour cream contain 3.1 grams of fat and 10 milligrams of cholesterol. Obviously, these full-fat dairy foods are not health healthy foods and should be avoided or eaten in very modest amounts.

Ice cream (another of my favorites) is also high in saturated fat and cholesterol. One cup of regular vanilla ice cream (11% fat) contains 8.9 grams of saturated fat and 59 milligrams of cholesterol! The fancy ice creams are even worse. One cup of rich ice cream (about 16% fat) contains 14.7 milligrams of saturated fat and 88 milligrams of cholesterol. Good substitutes are ice milk (3.5 mg saturated fat, 18 mg of cholesterol) and sherbet (2.4 mg saturated fat, 14 mg of cholesterol). Low fat frozen fruit yogurt is another good substitute for ice cream.

The Meat-Poultry-Fish-Eggs-(and Legumes) Group

The second part of the third tier of the Food Pyramid is the food group that contains the most calories, the most fat, the most protein, and the most cholesterol. It is an important food group for our health—and paradoxical too. Too little of this food group and we'd have protein malnutrition. But when was the last time you heard of protein malnutrition in America? Too much of this food group and we have high cholesterol, high LDL-C, high triglycerides, and obesity—followed by atherosclerosis, hypertension, diabetes and heart disease. It is a potentially dangerous food group. Typically, Americans consume too much heart damaging food from this food group.

Rather than continue to give it the long name in the heading, let's call this food group the Meat-Poultry-Fish Group (I'm including eggs as poultry). Most nutrition textbooks and government documents include legumes—dried beans and peas—in this food group. I prefer to consider legumes as a separate food group for reasons you'll understand a little later in the chapter. We could also call it the protein group because this is where most Americans get their protein—but that would be giving the incorrect impression that protein is not found in the other food groups. While this food group provides more protein than any other group in the typical American diet, significant protein is found in the Dairy Group, the Grain Group, and the Vegetable Group. Although legumes are considered a part of the Meat Group, they do not—unfortunately—play a significant role in the protein consumption of most Americans.

Meat, poultry and fish provide very high amounts of saturated fat and cholesterol. Let's look at some figures to illustrate this. In the lists I've provided here, I've selected some of the "worst" examples and some of the "best" examples based on the percentage of calories from fat. Corresponding information is also presented on eggs.

MEAT (3 oz cooked unless otherwise stated)

WORST EXAMPLES:

	Sat. Fat	Chol mg.	Total Fat, g.	%Cal Fat	Total Cal.
Beef:					
Chuckroast	9.3	88	23.4	68	308
Ground beef	7.8	76	17.6	64	246
Ground beef, extra lean	6.2	71	13.9	58	217
Top Sirloin	5.3	77	13.3	54	222
Bologna	7.2	31	15.6	83	170
Pork:					
Short ribs, braised	16.6	80	15.6	83	170
Bratwurst	5.6	33	14.2	78	164

BEST EXAMPLES:

	Sat. Fat	Chol mg.	Total Fat, g.	%Cal Fat	Total Cal.
Beef:					
Eye of Round	2.9	60	7.7	40	171
Processed lean roast beef lunch meat	1.2	17	3.0	39	70
Lamb:					
Leg, shank	3.9	77	9.8	47	186
Veal:					
Shoulder, whole	2.7	107 (!)	8.6	40	194
Pork:					
Ham steak	1.3	39	3.6	31	105
Loin, tenderloin	2.2	67	5.1	31	147

POULTRY (cooked unless otherwise stated)

WORST EXAMPLES:

	Sat. Fat	Chol mg.	Total Fat, g.	%Cal Fat	Total Cal.
Chicken:					
Leg with skin	3.2	79	11.5	52	199
Thigh with skin	4.1	79	13.2	56	210
Wing with skin	5.1	71	16.6	60	247
Turkey:					
Bologna	na	54	8.4	69	110
Hot dog	na	59	9.7	70	125

BEST EXAMPLES:

	Sat. Fat	Chol mg.	Total Fat, g.	%Cal Fat	Total Cal.
Chicken:					
White meat without skin	1.2	64	3.5	24	130
Breast without skin	1.2	72	3.0	20	140
Drumstick with skin	1.6	79	4.8	30	146
Turkey:					
Breast without skin	.3	71	.6	5	115
Leg without skin	1.3	101	3.2	21	135

FISH (cooked unless otherwise stated)

WORST EXAMPLES:

	Sat. Fat	Chol mg.	Total Fat, g.	%Cal Fat	Total Cal.
Finfish:					
Atlantic Salmon	1.1	60	6.9	40	155
Rainbow Trout	1.8	58	6.1	39	143
Anchovy canned	1.9	72	8.3	42	179
Pompano	3.8	54	10.3	52	179
Catfish	1.5	54	6.8	48	129
Shellfish:					
Shrimp	.2	167!	.9	10	85
Blue Crab	.2	85	1.5	16	87
Oysters	1.3	89	4.2	33	116

BEST EXAMPLES:

	Sat. Fat	Chol mg.	Total Fat, g.	%Cal Fat	Total Cal.
Finfish:					
Sea bass	.6	45	2.2	19	105
Swordfish	1.2	43	4.4	30	132
Orange roughy	0	22	.8	9	75
Tuna, canned in water	.2	25	.7	6	99
Atlantic perch	.3	46	1.8	16	103
Shellfish:					
Scallops	.1	47	1.1	8	125
Lobster	.1	61	.5	5	83
Clams	.2	57	1.7	12	126

EGGS

	Sat. Fat	Chol mg.	Total Fat, g.	%Cal Fat	Total Cal.
Whole egg, large	1.6	213	5.0	60	63
Egg yolk	1.6	213	5.1	78	59
Egg white	0	0	0	0	17
Egg substitute frozen, ¼ cup	1.2	1	6.7	63	97

Legend: Sat. Fat = saturated fat in grams
Chol mg = cholesterol in milligrams
Total Fat, g. = total fat in grams
%Cal Fat = percentage of calories that are fat
Total Cal. = total calories in kilocalories
na = not available

Source: National Institutes of Health, (1994). *Step by Step: Eating to Lower Your High Blood Cholesterol*. US Department of Health and Human Services. Publication No. 94-2920.

It is quite obvious from these tables that meat has more saturated fat and cholesterol than either poultry or fish, but that all three of these major protein sources for Americans are very high in fat and cholesterol. Before moving from this topic—the fat and cholesterol in this food group—I'd like to make my case for substituting the legumes for meat, poultry and fish whenever possible. Consider the table below—a comparable table to those presented above for meat, poultry, fish and eggs.

DRIED BEANS AND PEAS (½ cup cooked)

	Sat. Fat	Chol mg.	Total Fat, g.	%Cal Fat	Total Cal.
Kidney beans	.1	0	.4	3	112
Lentils	.1	0	.4	3	115
Pinto beans, canned	.1	0	.4	4	93
Black beans	.1	0	.4	4	113
Garbanzo beans/chickpeas, canned	.1	0	1.4	9	143
Black-eyed peas, canned	.2	0	.7	6	92
Soybeans	.6	0	5.6	38	117

(Source and labels as above except soybeans from USDA Home and Garden Bulletin #72, 1986.)

These numbers show that legumes have very low fat and no cholesterol at all (remember, there is no cholesterol in plants). They were included by the USDA in the Meat-Poultry-Fish group because of their protein content, so let's compare protein content by recommended serving size:

	Serving size*	Protein, gms
Meat	3 ounces	19-25
Poultry	3 ounces	16-18
Fish	3 ounces	11-16
Egg	1 egg	6
Dried Pea	½ cup cooked	7-8
Soybeans	½ cup cooked	10
Tofu	one 2½ X 2¾ X 1" piece	9

*Serving size recommended by *Dietary Guidelines for Americans.*
Soybeans and tofu data from USDA Home & Garden Bulletin #72, 1986.

The Table above demonstrates that dried beans and peas have approximately the same amount of protein as one egg, and about one-third to one-half of the protein found in meat, poultry or fish. The Vegetarian Food Pyramid places legumes (including soy products and peanuts) at the base of the food pyramid and urges us to consume legumes, grains, fruits and vegetables at every meal. I've included the Vegetarian Food Pyramid in Chapter 10, FAQs.

What is a meat-poultry-fish serving? The *Dietary Guidelines for Americans* recommend that we consume two to three servings from this food group per day. The recommended serving sizes are in the table immediately above. We must certainly choose carefully from this food group if we seek a heart healthy diet. Notice that 1 serving of meat-poultry-fish is 3 ounces—that's about the size of a pack of cards. Most Americans consume far more.

Excellent choices from the Meat-Poultry-Fish-Egg and Legumes Group. I think it is clear from the lists above that I favor the selection of dried bean and pea dishes, and the selection of lean poultry and fish over the selection of beef. Chicken and turkey without skin are good substitutes for beef, lamb, or pork products. Finfish is generally a good choice as long as hidden fats are not added (i.e., don't fry). Because of their very high content of cholesterol, I recommend the use of no more than two egg yolks a week. Egg whites may be used freely in cooking and in desserts.

Foods to avoid in the Meat, Poultry, Fish, and Egg Group. There are many foods to avoid in this food group. A heart healthy diet must be low in saturated fat and cholesterol, and meat-poultry-fish-eggs are generally high in both. Later in the chapter I will advocate an "almost vegetarian" diet, with only the most minimal use of red meat. Clearly, most red meats are high in saturated fats and cholesterol. Food preparation methods are very important to avoid adding hidden fats to poultry and fish, and make a big difference in the desirability of these foods. As a general rule, do not pan fry, deep-fat fry, cream, or use canned gravies or sauces with these foods. Chicken and turkey skin should not be eaten, and in fact, should be removed prior to cooking these foods.

Meat-poultry-fish-eggs and legumes are noted for their high protein content. But animal tissues are also high in saturated fat and cholesterol, and consequently, very careful selections must be made to achieve a Heart Healthy diet. Low consumption of red meat and higher consumption of legumes is recommended.

The Fats, Oils, and Sweets Group

At the very top of the pyramid, which means we should consume very little of these foods, is the Fats, Oils, and Sweets Group. The fats and oils consist of butter, margarine, lard, shortening, cooking and salad oils, and salad dressings. "Sweets" refer to candy and foods that are primarily refined sugars. Sweets should be avoided primarily because of their high content of "empty calories"—that is, foods high in calories (energy) but low in nutrient content. Candy and soda pop are examples of sweets with empty calories.

Although we don't "eat" the fats and oils as "foods" per se, we use them frequently in the preparation of other foods. Their use can significantly alter the heart healthy quality of foods from other food groups. Therefore, the selection and use of the fats and oils are quite important in a heart healthy diet.

Butter and lard are fats from animal sources, and consequently, contain cholesterol. Margarine and cooking or salad oils are fats from vegetables sources, and contain no cholesterol. (Note: Advertisements and labels on margarine and cooking or salad oils claiming "no cholesterol" are misleading, and silly at best. There never was, nor ever could be, cholesterol in them because they are derived from plants. Plants do not contain cholesterol. Cholesterol is found only in animal products.) There are other differences among these products as well. In the section on the Dairy Group, I explained that a fatty acid is a string of carbon atoms with hydrogen atoms attached and that it is the amount and way that the hydrogen atoms are attached that create different types of fat—saturated fat, unsaturated fat, polyunsaturated fat, and monounsaturated fat (see p. 133).

The use of these fats can significantly alter your total blood cholesterol and LDL-C. A diet that is high in saturated fat has repeatedly been shown to increase blood cholesterol and LDL-C. However, when polyunsaturated fats are substituted for saturated fat (holding total fat constant) there is a reduction in blood cholesterol and LDL-C (which is good) and HDL-C (which is not so good). This has been known for some time and is the primary reason why Heart Healthy diets have recommended the substitution of margarine (an unsaturated fat) for butter (a saturated fat), and the use of vegetables oils such as safflower, soybean or corn oils (polyunsaturated fats) for cooking. In the 1980s, however, studies showed that the use of monounsaturated fats could lower blood cholesterol almost as much as the polyunsaturated fats *without* causing a corresponding reduction of HDL-C, the "good" cholesterol. And, thus, many jumped on the bandwagon for olive and canola oils—oils high in monounsaturated fatty acids. Now, in the 1990s, attention has shifted to the "trans fats." A *trans fat* is a sort of hybrid fat somewhere between saturated and unsaturated. It is created when hydrogen is bubbled through a vegetable oil (an unsaturated fat) to cause some of the fatty acids to take up more hydrogens (to "hydrogenate" them) and thus make a liquid fat more solid. A semi-solid spread like margarine contains some trans fat. Hydrogenated vegetables oils are often used in commercially prepared foods such as baked goods and snacks. Trans fat has an effect on blood cholesterol that is intermediate between saturated fat and unsaturated fat—that is, it elevates blood cholesterol almost as much as does saturated fat, but not quite.

Heart Healthy diets substitute polyunsaturated and monounsaturated fatty acids for saturated fatty acids and trans fat. In simple terms use soft margarine instead of butter, use vegetable oils (particularly the monounsaturated canola and olive oils) instead of lard or shortening. It can get complicated, however, because fats and oils are more often a mixture of fatty acids as you can see from the Table below. The fats and oils in the table are listed from low-to-high saturated fat. Select fats and oils from the top of the list. Remember, all fats and oils are high in calories, and high in total fat. The bottom four fats and oils are known as "tropical" oils—note their high concentrations of saturated fat. Many commercial baked goods use tropical oils because they are cheap. Do your very best to avoid consumption of these oils.

COMPARISON OF FATS AND OILS

	Saturated Fat, grams	Cholesterol, milligrams	Polyun- saturated Fat, grams	Monoun- saturated Fat, grams
Margarine, diet	1.0	0	2.0	2.6
Canola oil	1.0	0	4.3	8.6
Safflower oil	1.2	0	10.6	1.7
Sunflower oil	1.5	0	5.7	6.5
Corn oil	1.8	0	8.4	3.5
Olive oil	1.9	0	1.1	10.4
Margarine, soft, tub	1.9	0	5.0	4.1
Margarine, liquid, bottled	1.9	0	5.3	4.1
Sesame oil	2.0	0	5.9	5.6
Soybean oil	2.1	0	8.3	3.3
Margarine, stick	2.2	0	3.8	5.3
Peanut oil	2.4	0	4.5	6.5
Shortening	3.3	0	3.5	6.0
Lard	5.2	12	1.5	6.1
Butter	6.8	28	0.5	3.3
Palm oil*	7.0	0	1.4	5.2
Cocoa butter*	8.5	0	0.4	4.7
Palm kernel oil*	11.7	0	0.2	1.7
Coconut oil*	12.5	0	0.2	0.8

* these fats and oils are used in commercially prepared goods.
(From Composition of Foods: Fats and Oils—Raw-Processed-Prepared, Agriculture Handbook 8-4, US Dept. of Agriculture, 1990)

What is a fat and oil serving? A serving size for this food group is 1 tablespoon which is about 120 calories—yes, wow! Remember, a fat or oil is 100% fat—9 calories per gram.

Excellent choices from the Fats and Oils Group. Choose fats and oils from the top of the table—those that are low in saturated fat and high in either the polyunsaturated or monounsaturated fats. Notice that there are four entries on the table for margarine. Diet margarine is manufactured so that carbohydrates are substituted for some of the fat content. It is lower in calories because it is lower in total fat content. An unsaturated fat tends to be liquid at room temperature—such as vegetable oil—and is far less harmful to your heart. Therefore, soft tub margarine and liquid bottled margarine have less saturated fat and more polyunsaturated fat than stick margarine. Stick margarine will have more trans fat than tub or liquid margarine. I recommend you use canola oil (high in monounsaturated fat) or safflower oil (high in polyunsaturated fat) for cooking oil. I recommend olive oil (high in monounsaturated oil) for salad oil because it is healthful—and tasty.

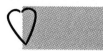

Fats and oils are heart damaging foods if used to excess. So are excessive sweets. Choose polyunsaturated or monounsaturated fats and oils for food preparation and salads. Limit sweets—they contain empty calories, and contribute to a sharp elevation in insulin.

Foods you should avoid from the Fats and Oils Group. For the reasons stated above, you should avoid the fats and oils at the bottom of the list—those high in saturated fat. These fats are potentially heart damaging foods. You need to be particularly careful in your selection of commercially prepared baked goods—in fact, I recommend you eliminate them completely and bake your own. But if that is unreasonable, then be sure to read the food labels and select baked goods that do not use the tropical oils. Look for use of safflower, corn or soybean oils. Avoid all foods that use lard or shortening, or palm kernel or coconut oils.

For a summary of the nutrients in each food group, see Appendix F, Nutrient profile of food groups.

READING FOOD LABELS

An important part of increasing your food awareness is the important skill of reading a food label. To make good food choices while shopping it is imperative that you read the NUTRITION FACTS on the government required food labels. Some parts of the label are very easy to understand...others are not so easy. Consult Figure 8.2. the food label from a package of frozen Fettucini Alfredo. Let's use this to consider the essential elements of reading a food label using the guidelines published by the Center for Science in the Public Interest.

1. Check the serving size just below the heading. Obviously, if you eat more or less than what's listed, you'll have to adjust the other numbers. The new food labels have more realistic serving sizes than in earlier years.

2. Next, check the column that is marked _% Daily Value_. This tells you how much of a day's worth of the nutrients listed the food provides. In our example, Total Fat is 36 g (grams) which is 56% of your daily fat limit (Daily Value). I recommend the following rule of thumb: if a food has 20% or more of the Daily Value, consider it "high" in that nutrient. If it contains 5% or less, consider it "low" in that nutrient. Remember, you eat 15 to 20 foods every day, so you don't want a particularly high percentage of any one nutrient in only one food.

3. Then check the % Daily Value for Saturated Fat and Cholesterol. These are the nutrients that are probably the most dangerous for your heart. Unfortunately, trans fat isn't counted in the food label. So if the food contains partially hydrogenated oils, the label will underestimate how much it may raise your cholesterol.

4. Then consider the _Calories_ line. The first number is the total calories in one serving. The second number is the number of

FIGURE 8.2
Nutrition Facts

Nutrition Facts

Serving Size 1 cup (249g)
Servings per Container about 2½

Amount per Serving
Calories 500   Calories from Fat 330

                                    %Daily Value

Total Fat 36g	56%
Saturated Fat 22g	100%
Cholesterol 110mg	35%
Sodium 910 mg	37%
Total Carbohydrate 33g	11%
Dietary Fiber 3g	13%
Sugars 5g	
Protein 12g	

Vitamin A 0%	•	Vitamin C 0%	
Calcium 20%	•	Iron 6%	

• Percent Daily Values are based on a 2,000 calorie diet.
  Your daily values may be higher or lower depending on
  your calorie needs.:

		Calories	2,000	2,500
Total Fat	Less than		65g	80g
Sat Fat	Less than		20g	25g
Cholesterol	Less than		300mg	300mg
Sodium	Less than		2,400 mg	2,400 mg
Total Carbohydrate			300g	375g
Fiber			25g	30g

Calories per gram:
Fat 9   •   Carbohydrates 4   •   Protein 4

calories from fat. In the example, total calories is 500, and the calories from fat is 330—that's 66 percent of the total. That's obtained by dividing the calories from fat (330) by the total calories (500) This Fettucini Alfredo is 66% fat—it is loaded with fat, and I'd classify it as a heart damaging food.

Percent of calories from fat = $\dfrac{\text{calories from fat}}{\text{total calories}}$

5.   Next, consider the *Total Carbohydrate* information. *Dietary fiber* is listed here as well as *Sugars*. Unfortunately, the Sugars number isn't very precise. It includes naturally occurring fruit and milk sugars, but it omits some of the "complex" sugars that are so important. The fiber number is quite important because you should choose foods high in fiber.

6.   The rest of the label allows you to compare the percent of Daily Value for "good" nutrients—Vitamins A and C, Calcium, Iron, and Dietary Fiber—with "bad" nutrients—Total Fat, Saturated Fat, Cholesterol, and Sodium. A heart healthy food should be high in good nutrients and low in bad nutrients—this one's a loser.

7.   The lowest part of the label is the same on all foods—so it tells you nothing about the food you are examining. This section gives you the recommended daily amounts for each nutrient for two calorie levels. Most of you will not be consuming 2500 calories, so look carefully at the 2000 calorie level. Adjust these numbers downward if you consume less than 2000 calories (and many of you do). Also, adjust these numbers downward if you wish to eat less than the standard 30% of calories from fat.

Debunking the Manufacturer's Labels

One of the best features of the new NUTRITION FACTS labels required by the U.S. Food and Drug Administration (USFDA) is that manufacturers must now comply with precise word definitions. The 1994 food labelling law brought order to what had become an advertising free-for-all. Terms like "low," "free" or "high" had long been used on food labels, many times duping the buyer to buy a product that was little different from the "regular" product. Such descriptions must now meet legal definitions.

This means that a food described as "high" in a particular nutrient must contain 20% or more of the Daily Value for that substance. So if you buy a bottle of fruit juice labelled "high in vitamin A" you can rest assured the product really is a good source of that nutrient. Unfortunately, some descriptors used on labels—the front side—can still be confusing. Here's why.

"Light" means half the fat, or one-third fewer calories than its regular version; it may also mean the sodium content has been lowered by 50%; or it may mean the product is low in fat or low in calories. The manufacturer is supposed to state the change or improvement in percentage terms somewhere on the package—so look for that. Light may also describe the color or texture of a food (for example, "light brown sugar" or "light and fluffy" cheese souffle.

"Reduced fat" means the product must have at least 25% less fat or saturated fat or cholesterol than the regular food. For example, a "reduced fat hot dog" must have at least 25% fewer grams of fat than a regular hot dog.

"Fat free" means there is less than ½ gram of fat per serving.

"Low fat" means no more than 3 grams of total fat per serving, and no more than 30% of calories from fat. In most cases, however, I wouldn't call a product with 30% of calories from fat, a low fat product. So, beware!

"Saturated fat free" means there is less than ½ gram of saturated fat in a serving, and less than 1% or less of total fat can be trans fat. This would be a good label to watch for.

"Low saturated fat" means no more than 1 gram of saturated fat and 15% fewer calories than the regular food product.

"Lean" or "extra lean" may be used to describe the fat content of meat, poultry, fish or shellfish. Lean means the product contains less than 10 grams of fat, less than 4.5 grams of saturated fat, and less than 95 milligrams (mg) of cholesterol per serving. Extra lean means less than 5 grams of fat, less than 2 grams of saturated fat, and less than 95 mg of cholesterol in a serving.

"Cholesterol free" means there is less than 2 mg of cholesterol and saturated fat per serving.

"Low Cholesterol" means 20 mg or less of cholesterol and 2 or less grams of saturated fat per serving.

"Low calorie" means the product has less than 40 calories per serving.

"Sodium free" means there is less than 5 mg of sodium per serving.

"Very low sodium" means 35 or less mg of sodium per serving.

"Low sodium" means 140 mg or less of sodium per serving.

Despite the 1994 law, manufacturer's still try to dupe you. To be a smart buyer you need to watch for food label hoaxes that say, for example, that a product is 99% fat free. This claim is based on weight not calories. For example, an "80% fat free" hot dog is one in which water and protein add up to 80% of its weight. It is not that anything has been removed from this hot dog—only that water has been added. This hot dog, compared with a regular hot dog, has the same amount of fat and protein, but more water. Both the regular hot dog and this "80% fat free" hot dog derive more than 75% of their calories from fat.

I just rummaged through my pantry and came up with a can of 99% Fat Free Chili (Turkey Ranchero chili with beans). At least that's what it says on the front label—implying that this chili contains only 1% fat. And of course, that's exactly what the manufacturers want you to believe. The back label (the official USFDA Nutrition Facts label) tells another story. A serving (1 cup) contains 3 grams of total fat, 1 gram of which is saturated fat. Calories per serving equal 240, with calories from fat equaling 30. Not too bad—this product is 12.5% fat—basically an OK food, but it is not a 1% fat food. The misleading claim is based on weight...remember, fat is light for its size, lighter than protein or water.

EATING HEART HEALTHY FOODS

A Heart Healthy diet should be made up predominately of foods from the bottom two tiers of the food pyramid—the grains, vegetables and fruits. That's because these foods are:

HIGH — in fiber
   in complex carbohydrates
   in vitamins and minerals
   in antioxidants
   in phytochemicals and
LOW — in fat, especially saturated fat
   in cholesterol
   in sodium
   in refined sugars.

These characteristics makes grains, vegetables, fruits and legumes Heart Healthy foods.

Does this sound complicated? It's not! You can do it. Here's how.

RESOLUTIONS FOR A STRONG, HEALTHY HEART AND VASCULAR SYSTEM

The easy to follow "resolutions" below will guide you to Heart Healthy foods and away from heart damaging foods. There are several ways you can implement these resolutions gleaned from the Center for Science in the Public Interest, the American Heart Association, and the *Dietary Guidelines for Americans*. You may decide right from the start that you will conscientiously follow all of them—at once. You may decide you want to implement each one separately, possibly a week apart, eventually implementing all the resolutions. You may decide that you already follow some of the resolutions, and that you only need to implement those you have not already incorporated into your dietary lifestyle. Or, you may decide that there are some resolutions that you just do not want to do and implement only those that are both convenient and that especially appeal to you. I suggest implementing these resolutions from the top on down—in order—but you may decide to implement each of the resolutions in a different order. For example, you may decide to begin with the resolutions that you feel will be easiest for you, and then, once you are successful, implement those that will be more difficult. Research has not shown that one method is any better than another—only that you must establish a plan. You best know yourself. Make up a plan (personalize it) to implement these resolutions that is realistic and attainable for you.

> EAT AT LEAST SEVEN SERVINGS OF GRAIN INCLUDING
> THREE SERVINGS OF WHOLE GRAINS EVERY DAY.

<u>*Why*</u>*?* Because grains provide fiber, complex carbohydrates, vitamin E, vitamin B-6, magnesium, zinc, copper, manganese, and potassium, contain no fat, and are low in calories. Grains are wonder foods in terms of preventing or reversing heart disease and its risk factors. Regular consumption of grains will help lower your cholesterol, your triglycerides, your

homocysteine, and your blood pressure (if it is elevated).

How to do it. Serving sizes make this resolution easier to accomplish than it might initially appear. One slice of bread is one serving. So a sandwich is two servings of grain.

- ❤ eat whole grain bread instead of white, wheat, multi-grain, bran, French, Italian, rye, or pumpernickel—which are all mostly white flour even though their labels may not seem so. Second best are breads that list whole wheat flour *before* any other flour.
- ❤ eat whole grain breakfast cereals like shredded wheat, Grape-Nuts, Cheerios, Wheaties, or Total
- ❤ alternate the cereals above with bran cereals like Raisin Bran, All-Bran, or 100% Bran
- ❤ use hot cereals like oatmeal, Wheatena, Ralston, or Roman Meal
- ❤ use whole grain crackers like Triscuits or Finn Crisps
- ❤ select whole wheat pasta, couscous, kasha, wild rice or brown rice

---

**EAT AT LEAST FOUR SERVINGS OF LEGUMES—
BEANS, LENTILS, OR PEAS—EACH WEEK.**

Why? Legumes, like other plant foods, are high in fiber and phytochemicals that reduce your cholesterol, blood clotting time, and blood pressure. They are also high in folic acid (folate) which acts to lower homocysteine. Like the foods mentioned in the resolution just above, legumes reduce your risk of heart disease, cancer, diverticulosis, diabetes and constipation. Legumes are excellent substitutes for meat, poultry, eggs and other high protein foods. Vegetarians rely on legumes. In my opinion, legumes should be listed in the Grain Group, and many nutritionists agree.

How to do it. If you don't now use a lot of legumes you will be surprised at how many wonderful dishes can be made. I particularly recommend a book called *Lean Bean Cuisine* by Jay Solomon (it's listed in the RESOURCES section in the back of the book).

- ❤ cook at least one recipe that is based on legumes each week, and make enough for leftovers throughout the week
- ❤ add canned (and rinsed) garbanzo beans to your salads
- ❤ eat lentils, split pea, or bean soup for lunch
- ❤ use bean dips or hummus (made from chickpeas) as a dip or sidedish. Try some ethnic foods like Indian dal (made of split peas or lentils).
- ❤ eat bean burritos and salsa for lunch (no cheese or guacamole)

**EAT AT LEAST THREE SERVINGS OF VEGETABLES AT DINNER AND
ONE SERVING OF VEGETABLES AT LUNCH EACH DAY.**

> EAT AT LEAST TWO SERVINGS OF FRUIT AT BREAKFAST AND
> TWO SERVINGS OF FRUIT AS SNACKS OR DESSERTS EACH DAY.

Why? Vegetables and fruits are high in complex carbohydrates, vitamins, minerals, antioxidants, and phytochemicals. All heart healthy nutrients. In addition, a diet rich in fruit and vegetables provides plenty of vitamin B-6 and folic acid to lower your homocysteine level. Unfortunately, the average American consumes only about three vegetables (one of them white potatoes), and fewer than two fruits per day. About half of all Americans eat no fruit at all! This resolution is probably the easiest way to ensure that you get the minimum number of servings recommended.

How to do it. Although this resolution may sound difficult to accomplish, it is not difficult at all because serving sizes are quite small: only half a cup for vegetables, one cup of salad, one piece of fruit, or one cup of juice.

- ❤ steam or microwave green beans, asparagus, broccoli, or Brussel sprouts, coat with lemon juice, mustard, and a touch of oil—delicious!
- ❤ microwave a sweet potato or yam until soft inside—good not only as a dinner dish, but as a snack
- ❤ take fresh or dried fruit to work for lunch or as a snack
- ❤ keep handy bags of frozen fruit or vegetables in the refrigerator—use for lunch or snacks
- ❤ buy baby carrots—great for lunch or snack
- ❤ eat a salad with plenty of dark green vegetables every day
- ❤ lightly saute sliced onion, peppers, and mushrooms and serve over pasta, or stuff into a flour tortilla or toasted whole wheat pita, or add to a two-egg (one-yolk) omelet
- ❤ a cup of juice is a serving of fruit—orange juice or tomato juice is an excellent source of vitamin C
- ❤ a good rule-of-thumb is to make ¾ of your dinner plate vegetables

Following these resolutions will put you in compliance with the DASH diet advocated by the National Heart, Lung, and Blood Institute of the National Institutes for Health. (DASH stands for Dietary Approaches to Stop Hypertension, a very successful program.) There are two small differences in what is advocated here—a little more emphasis on legumes than in the DASH diet, and a little less emphasis on meat. The DASH diet was shown to significantly reduce hypertension, one of the major risk factors for heart disease. It's estimated that following such a diet will reduce risk of heart disease by 15% and stroke by 27%. Put another way, there would be 225,000 fewer heart attacks and 100,000 fewer strokes each year. WOW! That's a greater reduction than can be achieved by drugs.

AVOIDING HEART DAMAGING FOODS

Foods that are high in fat (especially saturated fat and trans fats), cholesterol, sodium, or refined sugar are considered heart damaging foods. The following resolutions are aimed at reducing the consumption of such foods. Most offer a heart healthy substitute.

> EAT NO MORE THAN ONE 3-OUNCE SERVING OF RED MEAT PER DAY. AIM TO BECOME "ALMOST VEGETARIAN" AND CONSUME NO MORE THAN 3 SERVINGS OF RED MEAT PER WEEK. SUBSTITUTE SKINLESS POULTRY, FISH, OR DISHES BASED ON LEGUMES.

Why? By reviewing the table of worst and best examples of meat (see pp. 137-139) you'll see that meat, especially red meat, contains a high amount of fat, saturated fat, and cholesterol. This resolution provides a means to substitute high fat and cholesterol meats with other high protein foods that are much lower in fat and cholesterol. Several well known experts advocate vegetarian diets that do not allow you to eat meat at all. Dr. Dean Ornish's successful program for reversing heart disease is one of these. I highly recommend you read his book (it's listed in the RESOURCES section). Another is Nathan Pritikin's diet for increased longevity. I advocate a position in-between these rather extreme approaches. Although a vegetarian diet is very healthful—that's certainly what all research shows—it is probably not for everyone. I believe an "almost vegetarian" diet is the best possible substitute, and that an almost vegetarian diet is a very reasonable goal for most Americans. An almost vegetarian diet makes meat a minor part of the diet, and grains, legumes, vegetables and fruits a major part of the diet. The resolutions here are aimed at gradually easing you into an almost vegetarian diet. Aim to make other foods—not meat—the main stable of a meal.

How to do it. It's not hard at all.

- ❤ substitute meatless veggieburgers, Gardenburgers or ground turkey breast for your ground beef dishes (including "hamburgers") and hot dogs
- ❤ for meatloaf, meatballs, chili, or spaghetti sauce substitute chunks of meatless Harvest Burgers, firm tofu, or textured vegetable protein
- ❤ at fast food restaurants, select a grilled chicken sandwich (without mayo) or a veggi or chicken wrap or pita instead of a burger. If you must have a burger, select the smallest one available and hold the mayo and cheese

- as mentioned above—buy a good vegetarian cookbook (see the RESOURCES section) and try meatless main dishes based on soy protein. You're bound to find some exciting and healthful dishes that will surprise you with their tastiness. Be adventurous!

- substitute turkey bacon, low fat ham, or low fat sausage for your customary morning bacon (Healthy Choice, Oscar Mayer, Hormel are some brands to look for)—be sure to read the labels though so that you know exactly what you're getting.

EAT NO MORE THAN 2 EGG YOLKS PER WEEK.

Why? This resolution is aimed at reducing your consumption of cholesterol. Review the Table about eggs on p. 137. One egg yolk contains more than a full days supply of cholesterol if you are aiming for a total cholesterol intake of 200 mg. And, if you fry your egg or scramble it, the oil or milk you use may add even more cholesterol. Although some scientists believe that dietary cholesterol has little to do with the development of atherosclerosis, I'm not willing to take that bet.

How to do it. Remember that eggs are found in many prepared products—so even if you knowingly consume only 2 egg yolks per week, you are probably actually getting more.

- eat no more than 1 breakfast egg per week
- when you follow a recipe calling for whole eggs, substitute two egg whites for every 1 whole egg. For example, if a recipe calls for 2 eggs, use 1 whole egg, and 2 additional egg whites. You won't notice the difference, but your heart may.
- try egg substitutes (see Table on p. 137) but be sure to read the Nutrition Facts label. Although egg substitutes are low in cholesterol, they are higher in calories than eggs. If you also want to take off some weight, you need to realize that.

USE SOFT TUB MARGARINE RATHER THAN STICK MARGARINE OR BUTTER.

Why? Review the table comparing Fats and Oils (p. 141) and you'll see why. Butter is high in cholesterol and saturated fat. That's because it is a dairy product made from cream. Margarine is made from vegetable oils and therefore contains no cholesterol. To make a vegetable oil more solid, however, the unsaturated oils are hydrogenated. The end result is that stick margarines have more trans fats than soft tub margarines.

How to do it.
- ❤ just do it...use soft tub margarine
- ❤ try the lower fat tub margarines now available like Smart Beat, Fleischmann's Lower Fat, or Promise Ultra.
- ❤ if you must have butter, use a light whipped brand. You'll avoid several grams of fat per tablespoon.
- ❤ try Promise's trans-free spread (Fleischmann's product will be available soon)

USE SKIM OR 1% FAT MILK RATHER THAN WHOLE MILK, AND NON FAT OR LOW FAT YOGURTS. BE SURE TO EAT AT LEAST 2 SERVINGS EVERY DAY.

Why? Consumption of milk and milk products is important for women because we need a high intake of calcium throughout our lives to maintain strong bones and prevent osteoporosis. Postmenopausal women who do not use estrogen therapy should consume 1500 mg daily. That's a lot of calcium! The calcium found in dairy products is much more readily available for absorption from our intestine than is the calcium found in vegetables. So dairy products should not be eliminated from our diets. Whole milk is high in saturated fat (5.1 grams) and cholesterol (33 mg). So is whole milk yogurt. By switching to skim milk or 1% fat milk, and low fat or non fat yogurt, you will assure your daily consumption of calcium (in fact, it will be higher than when you consumed whole milk), and significantly reduce your saturated fat and cholesterol intake.

How to do it. Just do it.

EAT NO MORE THAN 2 OUNCES OF REGULAR (FULL FAT) CHEESE A WEEK. SUBSTITUTE LOW FAT OR REDUCED FAT CHEESES.

Why? Regular cheese (made with whole milk) is high in saturated fat and cholesterol and is our third highest source of atherosclerosis causing dietary fat (the first is meat, and second is whole milk). Reduced fat or low fat cheeses take a little getting used to in some cases, but contain significantly less saturated fat and cholesterol. So limiting your intake of regular cheese, and substituting lower fat cheeses will contribute significantly to reducing your intake of heart damaging fat. Next time you are in the grocery, read the labels and compare full fat with reduced fat cheese—you'll see what I mean.

How to do it. It's not so hard—even if you are a real cheese lover (like me).

- ❤ order your pizza with half the cheese and add lots of veggies instead (not meat)
- ❤ try the fat free cheeses (read the labels though, they add a lot of sugar). If you don't like them, try the reduced fat brands like Cracker Barrel ⅓ Less Fat (as a Cheddar lover, I like this), Jarlsberg Lite, or Borden Low Fat American.
- ❤ use "light" mozzarella in baked dishes
- ❤ order sandwiches without cheese saving your cheese servings for when they really count

> ADD NO MORE HIDDEN FATS TO OTHERWISE
> HEALTHY FOODS THAN ABSOLUTELY NECESSARY—
> LEARN NEW LOW FAT COOKING METHODS.

Why? Hidden fats may very significantly contribute to your total fat intake without your realizing it. A recent survey revealed that pan frying was still the most common form of food preparation in the U.S. If you pan fry a lot, be adventurous and explore new ways of food preparation.

How to do it. You may need to stretch yourself here to learn some new cooking methods. It's not hard though, and you may find out what foods really taste like when their true nature is not obscured by added fats.

- ❤ do not eat pan-fried foods, breaded (and fried) foods, meats basted with the fats that have dripped out of them (use a rack to raise meat and poultry out of the seeping fat)
- ❤ do not eat deep-fat fried vegetables, or potato and macaroni salads made with full-fat mayonnaise
- ❤ steam or microwave vegetables—add a little lemon juice and herbs and spices (no butter, margarine or cream sauce)
- ❤ braise, broil, roast or saute meats, poultry and fish
    - ♡ To braise, brown meat in its own oil (or add a trace of vegetable oil), then simmer in a tightly covered pan with a small amount of liquid (water, cider, dry wine, lemon juice, or a combination of these) until tender. Obviously, this is a wet heat method.
    - ♡ To broil, use a broiling pan or rack to allow fat to drain away. Use lemon juice or broth to baste. Most vegetables can also be broiled. This is a dry heat method.
    - ♡ To roast, bake in oven uncovered on a rack. This method takes longer than other methods. Add vegetables like potatoes, sweet potatoes, carrots, squash, or onions in the final 30 or 45 minutes. This, too, is a dry heat method.

♡ To saute foods, use a non-stick pan, dry saute (sear) meats and fish, then add a small amount of liquid such as water, lemon juice or white wine rather than oil. Vegetable broth can also be used. This is a wet heat method.

❤ use nonstick cooking spray rather than grease pans when cooking or baking

❤ remove skin from poultry before cooking

❤ make your own salad dressings

♡ Creamy dressings can be made with low fat yogurt rather than sour cream or mayonnaise. At least cut creamy dressings (such as ranch dressing) in half with plain nonfat yogurt.

♡ Use red wine vinegar or rice vinegar and you'll need less oil for a basic oil and vinegar dressing

❤ use mustard rather than mayonnaise on sandwiches

❤ use apple butter rather than butter or margarine on toast

> SELECT FOODS WITH LESS THAN 480 MG OF SODIUM AND AVOID COMMERCIALLY PREPARED FOODS.

Why? Not all people are equally salt sensitive, but most of us consume far more sodium than is healthful. In some people, lowering dietary intake of sodium (salt) will lower blood pressure by several points—enough to save about 10,000 lives per year from heart attacks and strokes. Most of the salt in our diets comes from commercially prepared or processed foods like soups, pizza, frozen dinners, lunch meats, hot dogs, and cured ham. This is one of the most important reasons you should make it a habit to read the NUTRITION FACTS labels on all the packaged foods you buy (canned goods, frozen foods, bagged or boxed foods).

How to do it.

❤ read food labels—become aware of high salt foods (more than 20% of Daily Value) in your daily diet (they don't necessarily taste salty)

❤ buy "healthy" versions of salt-laden prepared foods like soups, pasta sauces, and lunch meats. The word "healthy" can not appear on a label if the food contains more than 480 mg of sodium per serving. (For example, Campbell's Healthy Request Cream of Mushroom Soup contains 480 mg of sodium compared to 870 mg in their regular Mushroom Soup.)

❤ don't add table salt to the foods on your plate. Substitute lemon juice, ground pepper, herbs, or spices if you want to jazz up the taste.

> ### SWITCH FROM SOFT DRINKS TO FRUIT JUICE, SKIM MILK OR SELTZER.

Why? This resolution is aimed at reducing your consumption of simple sugars. Soft drinks are filled with refined sugar—each 12 ounce can has about 10 teaspoons of sugar, 160 calories, and—nothing else. This is a prime example of empty calories. (Only about 25% of our soda consumption is the "diet" type.) Statistics show that the average American drinks more than 50 gallons of soda a year. That's double the milk or coffee, and six times the fruit juice or tea we consume. But the danger is more than just high calories. A large intake of refined sugar causes blood glucose to rise sharply, and the pancreas must secrete a large amount of insulin to bring it back down. High insulin levels not only stimulate fat cells to absorb more fat, but make it more difficult for fat to be released for the production of energy by muscle cells. This leads to obesity. After years of high insulin levels, the pancreas may gradually become less and less reactive to high blood glucose—and insulin resistance develops. This can lead to diabetes, which as you remember from Chapter 3, is one of the primary risk factors for heart disease in women.

These problems with glucose metabolism do not occur with consumption of complex carbohydrates because they are digested much more slowly providing a very gradual release of glucose into the blood. This significantly reduces stress on the pancreas and lowers the risk of diabetes.

How to do it.

- ❤ select fruit juices, especially opaque juices like orange, grapefruit, tomato and prune juices because they contain more fiber than the clear fruit juices (apple, cranberry). Fruit juices provide vitamin C, folic acid, vitamin B-1, and phytochemicals. Healthy stuff—just watch the calories.
- ❤ if you need to reduce your caloric intake, drink flavored or regular seltzer or sparkling water. I like to combine orange juice with seltzer about half and half—it's zingy, lower in calories than straight juice, and more healthful than straight seltzer

I highly recommend you stay away from the diet soft drinks. The prime reason is that they "encourage" your sweet tooth. Another reason is that there is still some question about the safety of artificial sweeteners. Stick to healthy stuff.

> ### AND FINALLY...WHAT ABOUT THE NEW NONFAT OR FAT FREE FOODS?

Most of the resolutions in the section immediately above are directed toward lowering your fat and cholesterol intake. What about all those nonfat or fat free foods now available in the supermarket? Well, some taste much better than others. Many lack the "mouth-feel" of the regular food. Most manufacturers use gelatin or guar gum to add texture and thickness in an attempt to capture the "feeling" of the regular food.

You need to read the NUTRITION FACTS label very carefully on these foods. After all, if something significant is taken out of a food, something must be put back in...and you need to know what that is. In most cases, it's sugar, so fat free does not mean calorie free. Often, too, extra sodium is added to cover up the missing fat flavors.

Another potential problem with nonfat or fat free foods is that most people end up eating more than they usually would. They seem to lose any sense of moderation when they think the food is calorie free. So they eat a whole box of cookies at a time, or a huge dish of fat free ice cream when they would normally eat only a small dish of calorie rich ice cream. Research shows that people do this with artificial sweeteners too. Although statistics are not yet available on fat consumption since nonfat products became available, we know that the use of artificial sweeteners has *not* decreased the annual per capita consumption of sugar in the United States. In fact, it's higher than ever. I don't believe that the use of nonfat or fat free foods will reduce Americans consumption of fat either. More likely, caloric consumption will actually increase. I am much more in favor of consuming natural high fiber, low fat foods—and there are many of them we aren't accustomed to—than using nonfat or fat free substitutes of the same old foods we use on a regular basis.

You've probably heard of olestra—a fat substitute made from sugar and vegetable oil. It's becoming readily available—especially in potato chips. However, there are some real dangers with consumption of olestra, and I do not recommend it at all. Apparently the problem is that olestra interferes with the absorption of vitamins A, D, E, and K. Side effects include intestine and bowel problems such as cramping, gas, diarrhea, and "anal leakage." I wouldn't call that "healthy."

This has been a long chapter with lots of information to help you develop an eating lifestyle that is heart healthy. Together with daily aerobic exercise, a heart healthy diet will enable you to lower your risk of heart disease.

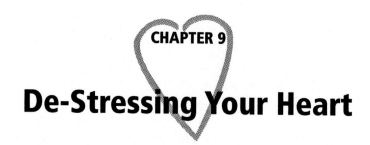

CHAPTER 9

De-Stressing Your Heart

There is no mistaking today, the importance of the mind-body connection in our physical health as well as our mental health. Descartes was wrong when he suggested that the body did not need the mind to function. In fact, *Descartes' error*, that the mind and body were totally separate, set medicine back years and years. Today, it is well recognized that the huge and complex system known as our nervous system—the brain, spinal cord, and peripheral nerves—controls our physical, as well as our mental, well-being.

It is increasingly clear that the way in which we perceive ourselves and the way in which we cope with daily life, very much affects the way our body works, and the way our cells interact with each other within our body. According to Dr. Herbert Benson, author of *The Relaxation Response* and *Timeless Healing*, our brain does this by responding to and interpreting messages from three different sources: our exterior environment, our own body cells, and the thought centers of the brain itself. The brain then retains a memory of every event and may (or may not) attach a meaning to that event. In fact, that is how we learn things like not touching a hot stove a second time.

In this way our brain "knows" who we are by transmitting signals to and from our body's cells and by incorporating our thoughts and imagination into the process. Thus, every event affects every other event. Exactly how our nervous system affects our bodily responses depends largely on what the brain "remembers." Many times this is good, but sometimes this is bad. Learning not to touch a hot stove burner is obviously "good." But learning that walking into a room full of people is stressful and developing a stomach ache because of that stressful perception, is "bad."

What the brain remembers depends largely on how we view ourselves relative to our environment, that is, the "world as we see it." This is a unique function of our socialization, our life experiences, our culture and religion, and our upbringing. What our brain learns and remembers, gradually becomes our beliefs about ourselves relative to everything else. If we feel incompetent, inadequate, angry, fearful, unloved and alone relative to an event—it will be remembered, and we will respond accordingly, both physically and emotionally. If we feel in control, adequate, confident, loved and secure—that too will be remembered, and responded to accordingly. Our remembered feelings become our beliefs, our learned conceptions— or often misconceptions—about ourselves; the constant internal dialogue that goes on, and on, inside us. It is this inner dialogue that shapes us and determines our future experience with life's events.

Today, there is plenty of evidence that our beliefs about ourselves can be a major source of illness—but we are learning that they can also be used as a major force for healing and overcoming physical illnesses. The purpose of this chapter is first to explain how *stress* (for lack of a better term) can negatively affect our heart and vascular system and contribute to heart disease; and second, to show you how to gain control of your beliefs and memories to affect heart healthy behavior.

Let's look at how the *stress response* works.

THE STRESS RESPONSE

The stress response includes all the physiological and emotional reactions your body is capable of. These reactions (which I will more specifically describe shortly) are manifested by a *stressor*, which is anything that causes *stress*. Stress is hard to define precisely. Usually stress refers to a feeling of anxiety and/or tension (both physical and mental) that occurs whenever some demand upon you exceeds your ability—or your perceived ability— to cope. The stress response is your physical and psychological (emotional) reaction to a stressor. Your physical responses prepare you to fight or run away—the "fight-or-flight response." Your psychological responses include your thoughts and feelings, your emotional responses about the event, and interact with your physical arousal. Often they are negative thoughts and feelings..."I can't do this." "I'll never be able to do that." "Why does this always happen to me?" "I hate—this job, that person, this place." Sometimes they are positive thoughts—"I love this challenge." "I can do this." "This is thrilling." So, although stress usually has a negative connotation, stress can also be positive.

Excessive stress—too much happening, too many bothersome hassles, too much to do with too little time or energy to do them, too many people making demands on you—causes *distress*. You feel overwhelmed, exhausted, "stressed-out"—and your body responds in sometimes very harmful ways. Distress is detrimental to your health and well-being.

"Appropriate" or positive stress, on the other hand, is helpful because it motivates you to do your best, it helps you rise to meet challenges, it inspires you to achieve beyond what you would normally do. Sometimes called *eustress*, it arouses you too, but in ways that are appropriate to the level of demand placed upon you. Thus, these responses are not harmful and may even be healthful—like falling in love, or being challenged in a sporting event, or responding to the audience as a speaker or performer.

Physical Responses to Stress

The most evident physical or bodily response to stress is the fight-or-flight response. We've all experienced this. Ever had a close call while driving? or had someone really startle you in the dark? Your heart pounds rapidly, your breathing becomes shallow, you breakout in a sweat, your muscles tense, you may get a dry mouth and stomach butterflies. Your hands may tremble. These responses—all designed to help you counter a frightening and potentially life-threatening event such as encountering a saber-toothed tiger, a sudden attack on your village, running from a prairie fire—are orchestrated by your nervous system. Your brain activates your *sympathetic nervous system* (a branch of your autonomic nervous system that you have little control of) which in turn:

1. increases your heart rate,
2. increases the contractile force of your heart allowing it to pump blood more forcefully,
3. dilates your coronary arteries and the arteries in your muscles so that these organs receive more blood and oxygen,
4. constricts arteries to your skin and abdominal organs because they aren't needed immediately and blood can be directed elsewhere (such as your heart and skeletal muscles),
5. dilates your breathing airways so that you can breathe more efficiently,
6. releases glucose from your liver and lipids from your body fat so that you have plenty of fuel for your muscles and heart,
7. concentrates your blood increasing the stickiness of platelets so that your blood clots more readily in case you are injured. You are ready—to fight or flee—and to survive a potential disaster.

When all this happens, wow, you are Amazon woman! You've heard stories about mothers lifting cars off children, or pulling unconscious husbands out of burning buildings, etc. These stories are true. And the fight-or-flight response allowed it to happen.

Obviously, there are times in life when the fight-or-flight response is entirely appropriate, even essential. Unfortunately, there are hundreds of times in your life when the response is activated and it is not at all appropriate—when none of these physical responses are needed because you neither fight nor flee (at least not physically). You don't need the fight-or-flight response when you need to give a report at a business meeting, or when you are late for something you perceive as important and are caught in traffic, or your child has been hurt and you are waiting for the doctor outside the emergency room. You don't need the fight-or-flight response every time you are feeling overburdened or stressed.

The fight-or-flight response I've described above is caused by acute or sudden stress, and is activated primarily by the nervous system. But acute stress responses—whether severe and frequent or partial but nearly constant—eventually become chronic. Chronic stress responses are more likely to be mediated by the endocrine or hormonal system than solely by the nervous system. With chronic stress, the adrenal glands secrete high levels of cortisol—the hormone ultimately responsible for most of our chronic stress responses and often called "the stress hormone."

Chronic stress is lasting stress caused by economic difficulties, intolerable relationships, or prolonged bodily pain. All too often we live lives that are overburdened with things to do; people to meet, places to go, bills to pay; sick children, husbands, parents; jobs we don't like and are not well suited for; a marriage that isn't what you dreamed it would be; financial demands and insufficient funds; excessive demands upon our time, our skills, our attention; followed by more demands, and more, and more. Sound familiar? That's chronic stress.

Whereas the fight-or-flight response is a sudden response to an alarming stressor, chronic stress is less extreme, less noticeable, not particularly helpful to us, and in fact, can be quite harmful in the long run. Our fight-or-flight responses become "sit-and-stew" responses. With prolonged chronic stress we become "stressed-out" and exhausted. According to the U.S. Public Health Service, 6 in 10 Americans report at least moderate stress, and 1 in 5 report "great stress" almost every day. Negative moods of loneliness, restlessness, boredom, and anxiety are experienced by a substantial number of American adults. Depression is particularly common among women.

Chronic stress, often manifested by chronic anxiety, depression, bereavement, or hostility, has been linked to heart disease, hypertension, cancer, suppressed immunity, asthma, back pain, chronic fatigue, gastrointestinal problems, headaches, and insomnia. Chronic stress is also linked with high blood cholesterol, glucose intolerance, obesity, smoking, alcohol abuse, and physical inactivity—all well established risk factors discussed in Chapter 3 for heart and vascular disease. Let's take a closer look at how your cardiovascular system responds to stress.

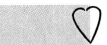

Acute or sudden stress stimulates the "fight-or-flight response" which enables you to survive an emergency or potential disaster.

Your heart rate increases, your blood flow pattern changes increasing the flow of blood to your heart and muscles. Your blood will clot more rapidly if you are injured, and you are suddenly stronger and able to fight or flee an enemy.

Specific Cardiovascular Responses to Stress: Fight-or-flight

Many of the fight-or-flight responses are cardiovascular responses—the pounding heart beat and changes in blood flow— that enable you to re-

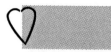

Chronic stress is persistent and nearly constant stress that stimulates the "sit-and-stew response" and leads to the physical or emotional exhaustion often associated with heart and vascular disease.

spond quickly to an emergency. The result is a sudden elevation in blood pressure. But this is somewhat different from the usual response to exercise in which there is an elevation in systolic blood pressure and a reduction of diastolic blood pressure. This occurs because the peripheral blood vessels open widely (dilate) during exercise to allow increased blood flow to your muscles and to your skin (for body cooling). During an acute stress reaction in which you do not actually fight or flee, however, both systolic and diastolic blood pressure rises. This happens because peripheral blood vessels do not dilate, and blood flow to your extremities is decreased rather than increased. Remember those cold hands when you are about to speak or present a report?

As long as you are totally healthy, there is no harm done and your heart rate will gradually slow, your heart contractions will return to normal strength, your blood pressure and blood flow will return to normal levels. These responses are the result of sudden and intense releases of *catecholamines*—chemical neurotransmitters released from nerve endings. However, to someone with a damaged, weakened, or unhealthy heart, such a sudden and high dose of catecholamines can be devastating. For example, a cardiac arrhythmia that interferes with effective circulation may be triggered. Or a spasm of a coronary artery may cut off blood flow to heart muscle. And thus, a strong fight-or-flight response can trigger a heart attack or cardiac arrest in someone so predisposed. And in addition, as acute stress becomes chronic stress, blood pressure remains chronically elevated—one of the most telling risk factors of heart disease.

Chronic Stress as a Cause of Heart Disease

When you are "stressed-out," your cardiovascular system is hard at work—continuously. Blood flow is redistributed so that, in effect, your blood volume increases. Your blood pressure (as explained above) is elevated, and your blood sugar, cholesterol and blood lipid levels are chronically elevated too. All these factors contribute to the development of atherosclerosis by causing damage to the inner linings of arteries (as explained in Chapter 2). In this way, stress can directly result in heart and vascular disease.

Research indicates that the chronically elevated stress hormones—the catecholamines and cortisol—also damage arterial linings and cause atherosclerosis. Coupled with the fact that blood clots more easily when you are stressed, there appears to be little doubt that chronic stress is an indirect cause of heart and vascular disease. More rapid blood clotting protects you if you should be injured, but with the sort of stress we are talking about here—the only injury will be to the interior lining of an artery, and increased clotting could be catastrophic by causing a myocardial infarction or thrombosis.

Chronic stress (as well as acute stress) may cause a sudden constriction of arteries already damaged by atherosclerosis. An arterial spasm caused by stress hormones may well be the cause of countless episodes of sudden cardiac death.

Chronic stress predisposes you to heart and vascular disease in other ways as well—it often leads to heart damaging lifestyle behaviors. People who are "stressed-out" smoke more, drink more, eat more (especially high-fat snacks), watch more TV, exercise less and are often either overweight or underweight. They also tend to use more drugs. Apparently they believe these behaviors enable them to cope better with job strain, feelings of incompetence, hostility, alienation, and hopelessness. At best, these behaviors temporarily distract them from the issues that are causing their stress.

STRESS, PERSONALITY AND HEART DISEASE

A controversial topic for years has been the question of whether or not there is a "coronary-prone personality." The so-called Type A Behavior characterized by an extreme sense of time urgency and a concern for high achievement was hypothesized to be coronary-prone in the 1950s. It turns out though that time urgency—characterized by nearly always doing more than one thing at a time (aren't most women required to do that?)—is not the essential element for a coronary-prone person, if indeed, there is a coronary-prone personality. In fact, time-oriented people often turn out to be quite well-adjusted to their level of stress, that is, they handle stress well, and appear to even seek it out. They love the challenge and get bored without it. Rather, the characteristic that seems to be most predictive of persons who have heart attacks—especially multiple heart attacks and sometimes sudden death—is that of hostility and anger. People who seem to have a cynical distrust of others also have chronically high levels of stress hormones and are "hot reactors" to aggravation. The *hostile Type A* tends to be in a nearly constant state of agitation—resulting in almost continuous overactivation of the fight-or-flight response. Unfortunately, not only are they "hot reactors," but they are also slow to cool down.

IF STRESS IS HARMFUL—IS PLEASURE HEALTHFUL?
THE PLEASURE/RELAXATION RESPONSE—
THE OPPOSITE OF STRESS

Too often we get stuck in the stress response—often with dire consequences—illnesses brought on by a chronic negative mental condition. Our body has opposing actions, however, that are an effective antidote for stress if we only learn to activate them. It isn't accidental that our body has a means to counteract the stress response. Nevertheless, for many reasons it seems that we often totally ignore that system—perhaps feeling guilty to even think about striving to experience pleasure. Often called the *relaxation response,* I believe it is more than that and so I'm going to call this the *pleasure response.* Let's examine the pleasure response to see how it counters chronic stress.

There are actually two branches of the autonomic nervous system—the system that is at least partially beyond our conscious control. We've already discussed the first branch, the sympathetic nervous system that is responsible for the fight-or-flight response. The second branch counters this response and is called the *parasympathetic nervous system* (PNS). The PNS inhibits or counterbalances the effects elicited by the sympathetic nervous system, and slows everything down again. It is the parasympathetic system that slows your heart rate after that scary emergency that stimulated the fight-or-flight response, and reduces the force of your heart contraction back to normal. It also helps to lower your blood pressure by redirecting blood flow from your skeletal muscles to your gastrointestinal tract so that you can digest that meal after all. It is the PNS that allows you to get that warm, comfortable feeling so familiar when you are relaxed and happy. It slows your breathing, relaxes your muscles, and lowers your metabolism allowing your internal perpetual-energy machine to ease down. Perhaps most important of all, the PNS lowers production of the stress hormones mentioned above—the catacholamines and cortisol. And when the PNS is stimulated you experience slower brain waves resulting in feelings of relaxation, pleasure, contentment, and rest.

Sounds wonderful, doesn't it?

Medical research tends to focus on the negative—the disease or illness model. I guess it's only natural—doctors are focused on making sick people well and have relatively little time left for what *keeps* people well, or on what nonmedical techniques such as meditation or prayer or even just plain positive thinking can do relative to healing. Things are changing though. With the rejection of Descartes' dual concept of mind and body, medicine (some people call this new trend Integrative Medicine) is beginning to examine more closely the interactions of the mind on the body and the body on the mind. And, as medical experts do that—considerable knowledge has emerged regarding how negative emotions detrimentally affect our health, and how positive emotions can heal us or keep us well. Some like to call this latter phenomenon the psychophysiology of pleasure (Barbara Brehm, 1998) or the biology of hope (Norman Cousins, 1989). Regardless of what it's called, there can be no doubt today that feeling good, being happy, experiencing pleasure, and knowing you're loved—contribute significantly to your physical health. Modern research clearly shows that happy people are healthier and live longer lives. And, they certainly enjoy life more than stressed-out people who are sometimes far too busy and distressed to even notice life around them.

If inducing the pleasure response is so good for us, why don't we seek it more often? Why are so many of us caught up in stress? One reason is probably because we've been so carefully taught the American work ethic that we believe that "wasting time" or "being non-productive" is bad. We've forgotten how to relax, we think it is "bad" to seek pleasure, we've gotten so out of the habit of smelling the flowers, of enjoying a sunset, of playing with our children, grandchildren or pets, of just listening to music—that we just don't do those things anymore. There just isn't time! We have too many other things to do!

I think there is another very important reason also—one that may be specific to women. We just don't think we are worthy to experience pleasure. We believe that instead of seeking pleasure for ourselves that it is our duty, our responsibility to deliver pleasure to others. And so, we become nurturers of others. As mothers and wives, we cook for others, we care for others, we are there for others—but we don't cook for ourselves, we don't care for ourselves, we don't nurture ourselves. We are so geared for others, we've ignored our selves. Although we may take the family on a picnic—we never simply take ourselves on a picnic.

And, when we do have some spare time, we fill the void with diversion rather than real enjoyment. Thus we watch too much television, we eat too much, we smoke too much (any smoking is too much), we drink too much (whether it's coffee, low-cal soft drinks, or alcohol), we work too much, and we exercise far too little. All too often we find ourselves in thankless jobs, thankless relationships that have lost meaning, and although we are busy, busy, busy—we are not feeling very good about what has become meaningless activity. Lacking simple pleasures, we feel empty inside—like something is missing. And it is!

HOW DO YOU KNOW IF YOU ARE CHRONICALLY STRESSED?

Everyone experiences stress. If you didn't I don't know that you could say that you were alive. We all worry occasionally about paying a bill, about the outcome of a medical test (our own—or someone else's), about a job interview or evaluation, or about the status of a relationship. We may get a stress headache or an upset stomach, or lose a night or two of sleep. We recover—completely—with no real side effects from this sort of stress. Although such stress may be annoying, it is quite inevitable—a part of life.

But chronic stress is something else altogether. It can be so insidious that we may not even know we are stressed. It occurs little by little, so gradually becoming a part of our lives that we may not even recognize that we are stressed. So how can you tell if you have chronic stress? Ask yourself the following questions—now I don't want you to be a hypochrondiac, but be totally honest with yourself. Don't exaggerate, but don't minimize everything either.

Physical Symptoms of Chronic Stress:

1. Do you feel tense much of the time?
2. Are you irritable much of the day? at home? at work?
3. Are you so anxious much of the time that you can't sit still to read? Do you feel jumpy much of the time? Do you feel hot (and sweaty) without probable cause (you will need to distinguish this from menopausal hot flashes)?
4. Do you suddenly find that you are late quite often—to meetings? appointments?
5. Do you often have difficulty sleeping? or fall asleep dead tire every night only to wake up in the middle of the night and then have trouble falling asleep again?
6. Do you feel tired much of the day? or lose energy at mid-day?
7. Do you have frequent headaches (that are not migraine)?
8. Do you frequently have tension or pain in your shoulders? or neck? or lower back?
9. How's your digestion? Do you frequently have an upset stomach? burp a lot after eating? have stomach acid or esophageal reflux? do you take a lot of antacids?
10. Do you have frequent constipation? or diarrhea? or gas?
11. Are you aware that you have a tight throat?

Psychological/Emotional Symptoms of Chronic Stress:

1. Do you feel fearful or apprehensive quite often?
2. Do you frequently become angry at work? at home? with friends?
3. Are you calm when you are have no control over a situation such as when stuck in traffic, or in a long line at the bank or grocery?
4. Do you find yourself becoming hostile when you are confronted by a stranger? your boss? a minority person? a person of authority?
5. Do you often feel like you don't fit in? that you are alone? that you are isolated socially? that no one understands you?
6. Are you depressed quite a lot? or continuously? Do you cry a lot for no apparent reason?
7. Do you frequently feel helpless to do anything about your life? your marriage? your family situation? your job?
8. Do you often feel hopeless? like there is little use to most everything you do?
9. Are you generally pessimistic about your future?

If you answered yes to several of these questions—and you are not just having a bad day—you are chronically stressed and in danger of poor health outcomes as a result. And, you need to do something about it. But before we get into ways to de-stress your heart, let's examine what I believe to be the primary cause of chronic stress in women.

THE PROBABLE CAUSE OF YOUR STRESS

Life moves fast today, and it is not always under our control. Dr. Dean Ornish, whose work I've mentioned previously has written extensively about how lack of real intimacy and feelings of being connected lead to emotional stress and heart disease. Many of us go through life with the perception that we are lacking something—that we are just not good enough. We believe that if only we had something we do not, then...everything would be alright.

- ❤ If only I had more money, then—
- ❤ If only I was prettier, then—
- ❤ If only I wasn't so fat, then—
- ❤ If only I was sexier, then—
- ❤ If only I was smarter, then—I'd be loved, I'd feel connected, I'd be happy, I'd be OK.

This feeling of being short on something, or not being good enough to receive something, or earn something, or accomplish something saps our feelings of self-worth. This lack of self-esteem is a matter of lack of self-love. Whenever we love ourselves so little that we find it hard to *like* ourselves, how can we possibly expect others to *love* us? And so we enter into a never ending cycle of not liking or respecting ourselves, feeling disconnected and alone, losing or never achieving intimacy, and feeling that there is something wrong with us—that we are lacking something others have. We believe ourselves unworthy.

"When we invest our self-esteem and self-worth in the outcome of an event or the behavior of another person, then we are giving that event or person power over our lives." (Ornish, 1990, p 101.)

According to Dr. Ornish, whatever promotes a sense of loneliness and isolation predisposes us to disease and premature death, and whatever promotes a sense of intimacy is healing. He claims that physical heart disease is emotional or spiritual heart disease, and that finding love and intimacy gives our lives a sense of joy and meaning. Perhaps John Lennon said it all when he sang "All you need is love." But to receive love and intimacy and a sense of belonging, you must first have a well-developed sense of self-worth and self-love. Before you can love others you must first love yourself. Before you can truly receive the love of others, you must first feel worthy. The rest of this chapter is devoted to achieving these objectives: first, self-love, then, extending love to others, and finally, receiving love and feelings of intimacy from others.

SELF-ESTEEM, SELF-WORTH, SELF-LOVE

Whether you perceive something as pleasurable, neutral, or stressful depends on how you conceive of yourself relative to your concept of the world. If you perceive something as threatening—whether it is physically or emotionally threatening—you will invoke the stress response. What is stressful to one person may not be at all stressful to another. The same event may be seen as an interesting challenge to one person, as humorous to another, and as an act of love to yet another. Whether you perceive something as pleasureful or as threatening is largely a function of your self-esteem, self-worth, and self-love. I believe this is particularly true for women because women are less likely than men to perceive of themselves as competent, strong (either physically or mentally), intelligent, creative, attractive, or lovable. Therefore, women are likely to feel threatened by an authority figure (a boss, domineering husband, father, or lover) and tend to react in a stressful manner to perceived dangers, to financial insecurities (bankruptcy, loss of job, loss of husband's job), family illness (whether child, husband, or parent), or conflicts with others (family, husband, parent, boss, child). The result is often stress-related disorders such as headaches, PMS, menstrual cramps, low back pain, heartburn, indigestion, irritable colitis, irritable bowel syndrome, heart arrhythmias, hypertension and obesity. Obviously, this affects your home and family life, your professional or vocational activities, and your personal and social domain.

If your perceptions are pleasureful, then you will invoke the pleasure response—and not the stress response. Your Heart Healthy goal is to spend some time each day in the pleasure response because it is an effective antidote for stress and stress-related illnesses.

COMBATING THE STRESS RESPONSE: INVOKING THE PLEASURE RESPONSE

There are many ways we cope with chronic stress. Coping mechanisms often serve to isolate us from the thing (or person) that we perceive as threatening. And sometimes that works very well. Other times, our coping mechanisms only serve to cause more stress.

A coping mechanism women use a lot is working hard. We are super-organized, we are super-mom, we are super-office manager, we are super-cook, we are super—everything. Some of this behavior is good, that is, we accomplish a lot and people think we are wonderful, and so we feel appreciated—sometimes. But much of this behavior is not good. We ignore our own needs. We spend so much time—at home or at the office—working to please others that we become invisible to ourselves. When that happens, we feel isolated from ourselves, and eventually we feel isolated from the very others that we are trying so hard to please. These perceptions lead to low self-esteem and stress—chronic stress. We are very likely to suffer health problems and perhaps not even know it until it is too late.

Other coping mechanisms are not very good for us from the outset—but again, we don't recognize that for some time. Eating too much is a common one. We eat to assuage our feelings of loneliness. We eat to make ourselves feel better—chocolate cake works wonders—only it doesn't really work for very long, and so we eat some more. Drinking is another coping mechanism used by many. Silent alcoholism (not outright drunkenness) is rampant in middle-aged women. Watching too much TV is still another coping mechanism. By plunging ourselves into the lives of soap opera characters, we can ignore our own plight. There are hundreds of coping mechanisms and of course, I can't mention them all here. But, you get the picture, coping mechanisms that allow us to forget about ourselves, that allow us to ignore ourselves, work temporarily, but not for the long run. If we fail to recognize that, we can end up with real troubles—feelings of isolation and chronic stress that may lead to heart disease or one or more of its major risk factors.

The procedures described below are designed to do several things. First, they are designed to quiet your mind—that's the specific purpose of the breathing exercises and basic meditation practice. Second, they are designed to enhance your concepts of self-esteem, self-worth, and self-love. That's the primary reason for the techniques to develop lovingkindness. Third, they are designed to allow you—in time—to reach out to others without losing yourself as so many of us have. Without a quiet and accepting mind and a strong concept of yourself in an external world, you can not really reach out to others to either receive their love or give them love without losing yourself. These procedures and practices will enable you to eliminate chronic stress from your life and enhance your ability to invoke the pleasure response. Let's proceed with step 1—quieting your mind.

Quieting Your Mind

Follow your breath. Begin to quiet your mind with special breathing techniques. First, simply observe your breath. This is a subtle and powerful form of breathwork that is very simple to do. You may sit or lie down comfortably with your back straight. Focus your attention on your breathing without trying to influence it. Notice that following your breath is pleasant and relaxing because it puts your mind in neutral. If your mind starts to wander—and it will eventually—just gently bring yourself back to your breathing. Practice this technique at least 5 minutes each day. Anytime is a good time. In addition, practice the technique whenever you feel stressed or anxious—but not when you drive your car.

The Relaxing Breath. This yoga-derived technique is advocated by Dr. Andrew Weil who teaches it to all his patients. It produces a pleasant altered state that feels better and better with regular practice. Here is how Dr. Weil describes the Relaxing Breath technique:

1. Sit or lie comfortably with your back straight. Place your tongue in the yogic position. To do this touch the tip of your tongue to the back of your upper front teeth and slide it back until it rests on the ridge of tissue between your teeth and palate. Keep your tongue there for the duration of the exercise.
2. Exhale completely through your mouth making an audible whoosh sound.
3. Close your mouth lightly. Inhale through your nose quietly to the count of 4.
4. Hold your breath for the count of 7 keeping the same cadence. How long you can hold your breath comfortably determines the rate at which you count.
5. Exhale audibly through your mouth to the count of 8.
6. Repeat steps 3 through 5 three more times for a total of four cycles. Then breathe normally and observe how your body feels.

The key is the 4-7-8 count cycle. Your exhalation is twice as long as your inhalation. Practice this technique twice a day. The best times are when you first awake and before you go to sleep, or just before mediating (this technique to follow). After you have practiced for a month, increase the breath cycles to eight.

When you breathe abdominally, you use your respiratory system most effectively. You should feel your belly expand when you take a breath in, and then return to normal when you exhale. If you are not sure that you are breathing abdominally, place a hand over your abdomen as you breathe. When you inhale your hand should move outward. When you exhale your hand should move back. If your chest rises as you breathe in and out, you are not breathing abdominally. People with asthma or other pulmonary problems often breathe with chest action and not abdominally. Many women have learned to breathe with chest action because they are so concerned with holding their stomachs in, and not looking fat.

Basic meditation practice. The technique made famous by Dr. Herbert Benson in his 1975 book _The Relaxation Response_, is a very simple and straight-forward technique for invoking the pleasure-relaxation response. It does not require extensive training, it takes only 10 to 20 minutes each day, and can be performed just about anywhere you can sit quietly without disruption.

1. Sit quietly in a comfortable position.
2. Close your eyes.
3. Relax all your muscles, starting with your feet and moving slowly up to your face. Keep them relaxed.
4. Breath slowly through your nose. Each time you breath out, say the word _one_ to yourself.

5. Continue for 10 to 20 minutes. You may open your eyes to check the time, but do not set an alarm. When you finish, sit quietly for several more minutes, at first with your eyes closed. Then open your eyes, shift your position around a little, and slowly stand up.

Do not worry about achieving a deep level of relaxation. Simply maintain a passive attitude and permit relaxation to occur at its own pace. When distracting thoughts occur—and they will—don't dwell on them. Just return to repeating *one* (*om*, if you prefer) with each breath. Use this technique once or twice each day. Digestive processes seem to interfere and so it is best to practice this technique no sooner than 2 hours after a meal.

Obviously, using this technique once or twice a day requires an ongoing commitment of time and effort. Believe me, it works wonders, so make the decision to do this and you will reap numerous rewards.

A word of warning. There is no right way or wrong way to meditate. You may well find that you can't seem to "stay on target"—observing your breath and saying *one*. You will have all sorts of thoughts. Trying to control the uncontrollable will simply lead to extreme frustration because most often you simply can not control your thoughts. The technique, although it sounds very simple, is not. Do not think of yourself as a failure if you just can not shut off your thinking process. Rather, the art of skillful meditation is the ability to let go and begin again—over and over and over. It does not matter that you need to begin again a thousand times during a meditation session. As soon as you realize that you are lost in thought, just stop, and begin again. There is no such thing as failure (although that is sometimes hard to believe). Meditation is simply learning to let go of distractions—your thoughts—and beginning again. That is the essence of mediation practice. So you see, not getting it is part of the practice.

I can't emphasize enough the importance of basic meditation practice. Meditation is the process of quieting your mind. This is done by paying attention, by increasing your awareness, by being in the present, by focusing on your breath. All this is called *mindfulness*. Mindfulness is paying attention to the present without judging and without preconceptions. Mindfulness means being totally aware of the present moment. When you are mindful of your breathing you are mindful of the present moment. As time progresses you will lose your sense of separateness and isolation and become mindful of the present. As you do that you will stimulate the parasympathetic nervous system, your stress hormone levels will be lower, and your brain waves will slow resulting in pleasure, relaxation, contentment, and deep rest. I promise you that.

For a more in-depth understanding of meditation and the pleasure/ relaxation response, I highly recommend that you read Benson's *The Relaxation Response* and Jon Kabat-Zinn's *Wherever You Go There You Are*. They are both national best sellers and will be easy to find in bookstores.

Developing Lovingkindness: Yourself

Self-esteem refers to your self-regard, your general sense of self-worth. Your perception of yourself relative to the demands you are facing determines whether you interpret the demands as stressors or not. In turn, your perception of your ability to cope effectively influences your appraisal of yourself—and so you have the cyclic problem mentioned earlier. When you develop respect for yourself, then you will be able to handle stress quite competently, and invoke the pleasure response quite often.

Self-esteem is directly related to your ability to cope effectively with stress. People with low self-esteem feel powerless and have a fatalistic view of life. They believe they can't control their lives which leads to a downward spiral—they expect to fail, and therefore they do. That, in turn, confirms their poor opinion of themselves.

A healthy self-esteem is based on loving but accurate self-assessment. Don't confuse this with egotism, self-centeredness, or snobbishness. People with these characteristics actually have fragile egos and are easily hurt. Consequently, they experience a lot of stress—and usually poor coping skills. Rather, a healthy and accurate view of yourself comes from accepting yourself as you are—right now, in the present—whether there are current problems or not. This leads to the confidence needed to confront and solve the difficult problems of life.

This step of the heart healthy program to de-stress your heart begins with learning to love yourself—with all your quirks and blemishes. You need to fully believe that you are worthy because of your uniqueness and the potential you hold inside. You need to believe that the basic spirit inside you is good, kind, loving, and lovable. You need to believe that your worthiness is not based on your accomplishments—no matter how wonderful or minimal they are. You need to develop unconditional self-love and self-worth. Begin by changing your self-talk, your critical self-talk.

<u>Changing critical self-talk</u>. Changing your self-esteem begins by changing the messages you receive, experiences you have, and ideas you form about yourself. When you take control of those messages, then you become the gatekeeper for the information you allow yourself to accept about yourself.

We all have a monologue running through our heads (did you think you were the only one?). Much of the monologue interprets and judges everything around us—and particularly, our behaviors and attitudes about what happens to us—spewing out commentary on everything. Self-talk is often based on our misconceptions about ourselves, and particularly about ourselves relative to others. It often represents irrational beliefs.

Dr. Barbara Brehm, in a book called *Stress Management: Increasing Your Stress Resistance*, reveals some common irrational beliefs many of us have:

1. It is an absolute necessity for an adult to have love and approval from peers, family, and friends.
2. You must be unfailingly competent and almost perfect in everything you do.
3. Good relationships are based on mutual sacrifice and a focus on giving.
4. There is a perfect love, a perfect relationship.
5. It is bad or wrong to be selfish.

Do these strike a chord with you? Can you think of others not listed here? Can you see how having these beliefs contribute to stress and critical self-talk?

Let's examine a couple of these irrational beliefs, and revise them into more reasonable and acceptable beliefs. Beliefs that will not inevitably cause us stress and negative self-talk.

Irrational belief: It is an absolute necessity for an adult to have love and approval from peers, family, and friends.

Revision: I want my peers, family, and friends to love me and approve of the things I do, but I realize that I can't always please everyone all the time. I will do my best, do what I feel in my heart is right, and accept the fact that not everyone will always agree with me.

Now won't this be an easier expectation to live with than the irrational belief?

Irrational belief: You must be unfailingly competent and almost perfect in everything you do.

Revision: I will do my best and learn from my mistakes.

Think of all the irrational beliefs you have—and write revisions of them that are reasonable and that you can live comfortably with.

Our irrational beliefs result in terribly negative self-talk because we simply can not live up to these beliefs. Whenever you realize you are engaging in negative self-talk do two things:

First, say to yourself. "Oh, woe is me" (or something to that effect) to lighten your mood a little, and draw attention to your negative self-talk. Then, of course, stop the inner talk altogether, or better yet, change it to positive self-talk.

Then, when time is appropriate, examine the irrational belief you hold about yourself that led to your negative self-talk, and revise it into a belief that is reasonable and livable. Be honest with yourself, but realistic. Above all, be kind to yourself.

The lovingkindness meditation: Self-love. This next technique is a major step in learning to combat stress and invoke the pleasure response, and shouldn't be initiated until you have been practicing the quieting your mind techniques for at least one month. Don't hurry this. I ask only that you read the material below now, but not attempt it until you have been following your breath, practicing the relaxing breath, and using the basic meditation technique for one month.

The meditation practice below comes from a book entitled *Lovingkindness: The Revolutionary Art of Happiness* by Sharon Salzberg, and is designed to help you further your self-respect and self-love—to develop lovingkindness toward yourself. After you have successfully completed this step, a similar meditation will be done to extend lovingkindness to others.

But first, what is lovingkindness? *Lovingkindness* is the ability to embrace all parts of yourself as well as all parts of the world. It means finding inner integrity because it relieves you of the need to deny aspects of yourself you don't like very much. When you are open to everything about yourself, you find the healing force of self-respect and self-love. With lovingkindness you realize that the mind is naturally radiant, pure and good. You realize that when certain negative states arise—such as anger, fear, guilt, greed, envy—that you lose touch with the fundamentally pure nature of your mind, and you suffer. Your challenge is to see these torments for what they are, brief and meaningless visitors that you need to acknowledge, and then move beyond. When you achieve lovingkindness toward yourself, you will not be shattered by stress. The force of lovingkindness will enable you to dislodge your anger or guilt, and return to your natural and good state of mind. Uncovering the force of self-respect and self-love will dislodge fear, anger, guilt, etc., and you can truly befriend yourself. Your tendency toward mental self-flagellation will disappear. Your self-hatred will no longer sustain itself. It is only when you see the goodness in yourself, that you will be able to able to focus on the positive, to seek pleasure rather than stress, and become impermeable to the sense of lacking that formally devastated your mind.

How to do the lovingkindness meditation: Self-love. In the lovingkindness meditation you gently repeat phrases that are meaningful in terms of what you wish for yourself. The aspirations you articulate should be deeply felt and enduring. You may come up with your own phrases, but the phrases classically used are:

> "May I be free from danger."
> "May I have mental happiness."
> "May I have physical happiness."
> "May I have ease of well-being."

Sit comfortably. Begin with a few minutes of reflection on the good within you or your wish to be happy. Then choose three or all four of the phrases above that express what you most deeply wish for yourself, and repeat them over and over again. You can coordinate the phrases with your breath, or simply have your mind rest in the phrases without a physical anchor.

Develop a gentle pacing with the phrases; there is no need to rush through them. Think of offering yourself a gift with each phrase. If your attention wanders, or difficult feelings or memories arise, acknowledge them and gently let them go in the spirit of kindness, and begin again. Remember, meditation is an exercise in beginning—again and again.

If feelings of unworthiness come up, simply accept that these feelings have arisen, breathe gently letting them go with your out-breath, and return to the phrases.

You can be creative with the phrases you choose to make them more closely fit your life and desires. For example, "May I be free from danger" could be "May I be free from fear." "May I have mental happiness" could be "May I be peaceful" or "May I be happy." "May I have physical happiness" could become "May I be healed" or "May I be healthy" or "May I embody my love and understanding." "May I have ease of well-being" could be "May I live with ease" or "May I dwell in peace" or "May lovingkindness manifest throughout my life."

If you have trouble getting started with this meditation imagine yourself sitting with all the most loving people you have heard of in the world—Jesus, the Buddha, Gandhi, the Dalai Lama, Mother Theresa—and receiving their kindness and good wishes.

Coming to terms with your body. Many women, perhaps even most women, dislike, even hate, their bodies. That's why so many of us are constantly trying to lose weight, or getting our hair done or recolored, or working on our nails. And indeed, appearance is not just skin-deep; it has a profound effect on your self-esteem and self-confidence. We all care what people think about our appearance—no matter what we may say about that. We are stung by criticism and empowered by praise.

One of the most intimate acts you can perform is standing in front of a mirror and studying your body. There, you will see things you like, and things you don't like. And so, building self-esteem and self-love would be incomplete if you did not focus some time on learning to love your body—as it is—in the present. If you can not accept your body as it is, it will certainly be difficult for you to feel worthy of receiving love from others.

According to George Leonard and Michael Murphy in *The Life We Are Given*, our posture is one of the most comprehensive statements we make about ourselves. To stand more erectly is to change your relationship with the world. And so, do this moving meditation at least once a week—to alter your concept of body and increase your body-love.

Find a quiet time when you will be undisturbed. Play some soothing, quiet music on the radio or stereo—something New Age, or mystical in nature—music without vocals or words that can be understood. Slow music. Darken the room some—maybe use candle light, and make sure the room is warm and comfortable. You may strip off your clothes or remain fully clothed—whichever you prefer. Maybe you will want to do this fully clothed a few times before removing your clothes. Begin by moving slowly around the room—to the rhythm of the music, slowly and sensually—this is not meant to be sexual in nature—you are simply to enjoy the movement of your body and experience pleasure from the movement. If you are inhibited, imagine yourself as a dancer who is practicing alone. Concentrate on the movement of your body and how competent it feels. Don't worry about how you look, or whether you are "doing it right," because there is no "right" way. Instead, just move slowly and steadily. Think about being beautiful—feel that you are beautiful. Enjoy each moment. Be beautiful.

If you begin to feel ridiculous, or awkward, or ugly—just as in sitting meditation, acknowledge the thought, breathe it out with a deep exhalation, and keep moving. Think beauty and flowing and being one with the music.

Developing Lovingkindness: Others

According to Dr. Dean Ornish (*Reversing Heart Disease* and *Love and Survival*), "the perception of being isolated is a fundamental cause of why we react to the world in ways that cause us to feel stress." Your heart health is as much about finding love and intimacy as it is about reducing your cholesterol and blood pressure. Ornish claims that whatever promotes a sense of loneliness and isolation—from yourself, other people, or something spiritual—predisposes you to disease and premature death. Whatever promotes a sense of intimacy is healing.

The meditation below, adapted from Salzberg's *Lovingkindness*, is an extension of the meditation technique described above. It is a natural extension of developing intimacy with yourself and allows you to achieve the power of connection—to others, and to all beings. The following is a three step process and will take some time to perfect (if indeed, we ever perfect lovingkindness)—perhaps years. When you feel that you have been successful with the lovingkindness meditation focused on yourself, begin to extend yourself with the following.

Lovingkindness: A benefactor. Sit comfortably. Spend a few minutes following your breath. Then, gently repeat the lovingkindness phrases you have chosen offering friendship and love to yourself. After about 10 minutes, bring to mind someone for whom you feel strong respect or gratitude—a benefactor or mentor. As you call this person to mind, visualize that person and recall the different ways he or she has helped you or contributed to your life. Recall the goodness within that person. Then, direct the lovingkindness phrases you have used for yourself to your bene-factor. "Just as I want to be happy, so do you want to be happy. May you be happy." Over time, the phrases you used previously may be altered to better fit your benefactor. Try to connect to each phrase, one at a time. Don't struggle to manufacture a feeling of love, simply repeat the phrases, and trust that the nature of your mind will take its own course.

Lovingkindness: A beloved friend. With this technique, everything is the same as above, but now you focus on a beloved friend. Begin by fol-lowing your breath. Then, reflect on the meaning of friendship to you. Af-ter about 5 minutes, direct lovingkindness toward yourself. When you are ready to do so bring to mind someone you consider a good friend, saying his or her name, bringing an image of that person to mind, or getting a feeling of the presence of that person. Direct the force of lovingkindness toward the beloved friend by repeating the phrases you have chosen for yourself. If the phrases change or if a different friend comes to mind, allow that to happen. If your mind wanders off to stories or future plans, gently return to the repetition of the phrases.

Lovingkindness: A neutral person. As you progress, you will eventually be ready to extend your feelings of lovingkindness to someone toward whom you have a completely neutral feeling. This should be someone who you have formed neither an instant liking nor disliking, perhaps someone you see only occasionally that you have no intense feelings for one way or another.

Reflect on that person's wish to be happy, and direct the lovingkindness phrases toward the person. If you feel bored, or distracted, go back to sending lovingkindness phrases to yourself or to a beloved friend, then, when you are ready, return to the neutral person.

In time, you will discover an increase in caring and warmth toward the neutral person. He or she will seem much closer to you—the person has become a sort of secret love.

Lovingkindness: Difficult persons and all beings. Eventually, the prac-tice of lovingkindness meditations should be extended to persons with whom you have had conflict (difficult persons) and to all beings in the world (to extend your concept of universal oneness), but these medita-tions are beyond the scope of this book. If you wish to truly extend your-self, I recommend you read Sharon Salzburg's book cited above, and a tiny book by Pema Chodron, *Awakening Loving-Kindness* (Shambhala Pocket Classics, 1996).

Combating Isolation

Sometimes, "All you need is love." A common source of stress today is isolation. Dr. Ornish believes that people who are lonely, depressed, and hostile are up to ten times more likely to have a heart attack compared to those who have love, companionship, and a sense of community in their lives. Think about it—we don't have community schools in the sense that we did 30 and 40 years ago. The church is no longer a primary center of our lives. Many of us don't know our neighbors. Some of us live in highrise steel and concrete fortresses. We drive the freeway to work, have a busy and stressful day, and then hurry home again on the freeway to—what?

If you feel isolated and lonely, you have chronic stress. A way to change this is to look around for something to do that will help make the world a better place. You need to reach out, because people will most likely not simply come to you. Here are some ideas:

Tutor a child. Join a neighbor group. Be active in church. Do activities related to a hobby (like birds? join a local birding group). Donate time to a theater or music group. Start a _____ group. Take an elderly friend shopping. Join a support group. Set some goals about reaching out and helping others (remember, personalize the goal, make it realistic and specific).

CONCLUSION

The purpose of this chapter has been three-fold. First, to alert you to the dangers of stress, and describe its probable cause. Second, to empower you to either eliminate stress from your life or to cope successfully with it. And third, to enable you to invoke the pleasure/relaxation response to find love and intimacy and a sense of connection not only with yourself, but with the outer world. All this is important because it is becoming increasingly clear that our mental and emotional attitudes toward ourselves and others, and how we cope with daily life, play an essential role in our heart health.

CHAPTER 10

Frequently Asked Questions (FAQs)

This last chapter contains answers to questions I've received over the years of working with people on fitness and health issues. Some are specific to heart disease, but many are not. All apply either directly or indirectly to women at risk for heart disease and heart attack. I've grouped the questions together by general topic. The first set of questions are about physical activity and fitness, with a subset about weight and dieting. The second set are about nutrition and dietary supplements, and the third set, are about stress-related topics. If you have questions I haven't addressed, send them to me and I'll include them in any second edition of this book.

QUESTIONS ABOUT PHYSICAL ACTIVITY AND FITNESS

Q: What about walking outdoors in winter?

A: Winter is a wonderful time for brisk walking. (You didn't think I was going to let you off, did you?) Depending on where you live, you'll have to be careful about ice. Snow slows you down, so expect to slow your pace. You'll probably also find that you'll have to change your regular walking shoes for something heavier. Usually a lightweight hiking boot will do, but be sure to pick one with good tread to give you some traction. Think of your walking boots as snow tires.

Some wonderful synthetic materials are available today that will keep you warm in cold or windy weather yet permit you to "breathe" so that you don't get soaked from sweating under your clothes. Nothing is more uncomfortable and dangerous than working up a sweat and then getting cold. These materials are designed for layering, a concept for dressing that was developed by people heavily into outdoor sports like backpacking, cross-country skiing, and mountain climbing. In those situations, dressing poorly can lead to life-threatening loss of body heat.

The *layering principle* refers to dressing in layers so that air pockets are created around your body. Air is an excellent insulating material—it just has to be trapped. That's the whole idea behind a goose down sleeping bag. It's not the goose down that makes you so warm (have you ever tried a goose down comforter? It's wonderful!); it's the air trapped by the goose down and the covering material. Applying this concept to sports clothing goes like this:

The first layer is a thin polypropylene (polypro for short) shirt next to your skin (it looks like a short- or long-sleeved T-shirt). I can't emphasize enough how important this first layer is. Even if you don't exercise hard enough to sweat a lot, we all have body moisture. The idea is to wick sweat and body moisture away from your skin. If, instead, this moisture is trapped next to your body, you will get chilled—I guarantee it! Don't wear cotton next to your skin in winter. It will soak up sweat and there it sits—next to your skin. You'll end up chilled. I recommend Cool-max™ as a first layer (a form of polypropylene). You'll find Cool-max shirts in some running stores, bike shops, ski shops, outdoor clothing stores, or sportswear mail-order houses like Early Winters or L.L. Bean. (I've never seen anything appropriate in a department store.)

The second layer is a middle-weight polypro shirt (for example, a turtleneck, long-sleeved crew-necked shirt, or a button-up shirt). Some attractive materials and styles are available now (used to be only black and navy).

The third layer is a heavier polypro fleece shirt or jacket. I particularly like Polartec™.

The fourth layer is a wind-resistant, water-resistant, breathable jacket that makes up the outside shell. Gore-Tex™ is an example, but many less expensive microweaves are now available. Ultrex is one. Ask salespeople in shops that specialize in outdoor sports apparel to help you.

Vary the middle two layers according to the weather. When it is warm, you use only the first layer. If it is windy and a little cooler you add the second layer. If it is windier and cooler yet, add the shell (the fourth layer), skipping the third. Use the third layer only on the coldest days.

> **Q:** What about swimming as aerobic exercise? I've always understood that it is one of the very best forms of exercise, but you don't mention it.

A: You're right, swimming is one of the best forms of all-around exercise because it requires the use of all the major muscles. Swimming, however, is a very inefficient exercise. It takes considerable effort to go even a short distance, particularly if you are not highly skilled at it. That means that you will become exhausted in such a short time that you will be unable to complete enough swimming to get the benefits you desire.

(I've known many women who have attempted to lose weight by daily swimming. They swam day after day, didn't lose much weight, and became discouraged. I think it was because they didn't swim fast enough. In their cases, I think they were comfortable in the water and swam very slowly.) Another reason I have not mentioned swimming is that we need to stimulate our bones (particularly as we enter and pass our 40s) to maintain our bone mineral mass and prevent osteoporosis. The best way to do this is with weight-bearing exercise. Swimming, of course, is *not* a weight-bearing exercise. When you are in the water, you are basically supported by it, and the stress and strain on your bones is mild.

But, having said that, perhaps the best way you can use swimming to reduce your risk for heart disease is to alternate it with walking. If you are good at swimming, and particularly enjoy it, why not use swimming as a complement to your walking? Some people suffer joint problems if they walk every day, and for them alternating swimming and walking is an excellent alternative. As implied above, swimming is much less stressful on the joints of the lower body than walking—but unfortunately, it is more stressful on the shoulder joints (ever hear of swimmer's shoulder?).

If you have a readily available place to swim, you might wish to walk three or four times per week and swim two to three times. The best stroke to use for fitness (and calorie consumption) is the front crawl stroke, but you can use other strokes as well.

To accomplish the purposes of aerobic exercise emphasized in this book, you need to practice long-distance swimming. Simply paddling around for a while won't do. You need to work up to swimming a mile or more at a time, and you should monitor your swimming intensity just as you would your walking intensity. Here's another advantage of the rating of perceived exertion (RPE) method (versus counting your heart rate). When swimming, your maximal heart rate is 13 to 15 beats slower than when doing upright, weight-bearing exercise. This is due to the effect of cool water and the horizontal position of swimming, which changes your blood distribution. The perceived exertion method accounts for this. So, as described in Chapter 7, aim for an RPE of 12 at first and then 13 to 14.

In swimming for fitness, you need to maintain a high enough cadence (stroke rate) to challenge your heart, lungs, and muscles. Leisurely swimming will not do this.

> **Q: My fitness club has a lot of stationary bikes—both upright and recumbent. Can I substitute stationary cycling for walking?**

A: Bicycling, and by that I mean road cycling, is an enjoyable and rewarding form of aerobic exercise. But stationary cycling? Fun? Personally, I've never known anything so boring! And you get so hot because very little air is moving around your body. In road cycling, air movement around your body causes sweat to evaporate immediately. Consequently, you feel cool. In addition, like swimming, cycling (whether road or stationary) is *not* weight-bearing exercise. Therefore, although you get more stress and strain on your bones (your leg bones anyway) than with swimming, you do not get the benefits of weight bearing on your spine, pelvis, and hips. I think that's important for middle-aged women, and that's one of several reasons that I've emphasized walking.

Yet another reason (not convinced yet?) is that most women find bicycle seats very uncomfortable. Because of that, they are unlikely to stay with a boring indoor cycling program for long. But if you wish to alternate stationary cycling with walking, here's a good way to do it.

Adjust your seat so that your legs are nearly straight on the down stroke (the six o'clock position) when your heels are on the pedals. Then place your feet on the pedals so that the balls of your feet (the strong part, not your instep) provide the pushing force. I recommend you use foot straps or toe clips. Next, choose a cycling resistance level at which you can maintain a cadence of at least 80 rpm for 15 minutes. Once you have established that, do the following 35-to 45-minute workout. You won't get bored with this. Vary the cycling resistance or your cadence (or both) to adjust your effort or perceived exertion (RPE). *Steady state* means that you have an elevated heart rate and breathing level, but you are comfortable and could sustain this level for quite some time. *Aerobic interval* means that you are pushing yourself—not to exhaustion, but to a level above steady state. During *recovery*, reduce the resistance so that you can bring your heart rate and breathing back down to the steady state level before your next interval. This workout is guaranteed to increase your fitness level.

	Duration (minutes)	RPE(effort)
Warm-Up	4-5	10 (light)
Steady state	5	12 (moderate)
Aerobic interval	3-5	13 (somewhat hard)
Recovery	2	11 (fairly light)
Aerobic interval	3-5	14 (somewhat hard)
Recovery	2	11 (fairly light)
Aerobic internal	3-5	15 (hard)
Recovery	2	11 (fairly light)
Steady state	5	12 (moderate)
Cool-Down	3	10 (light)

As I've emphasized before, have fun with this. You can do this workout on either an upright bike or a recumbent bike. For that matter, you can do it on just about any type of exercise machine.

Q: I keep hearing about cross-training. What does it mean, and should I do it?

A: Cross-training basically means that you do a variety of things (rather than only one) on a regular basis—like walking one day, swimming the next day, weight lifting the third day, and so on. Of course, there are all sorts of combinations. Some people will walk for 30 minutes and lift weights for 30 minutes for an hour of exercise.

Cross-training offers several advantages and I highly recommend it. One is that you are less likely to overstress any single part of your body and therefore are less likely to develop an overuse injury. Another is that you exercise all parts of your body—not just your legs and lungs (as I've emphasized here to benefit your heart). I believe that women over 40 should be lifting weights on a regular basis to protect their bone density and prevent osteoporosis (unless they do heavy manual work). Cross-training provides a system for exercising aerobically (walking or cycling or swimming or dancing), that is good for your heart, and doing resistance exercise (weight lifting) that is good for your muscles. Given the best of all worlds, I'd have everybody cross-training.

Instruction in weight lifting is beyond the scope of this book. I highly recommend *Weight Training for Dummies* by Liz Neporent and Suzanne Schlosberg to get started. Or join a fitness club and work with a trainer there.

Q: I have low-back pain that often flares up when I begin an exercise program. Do you have any suggestions on how I can prevent this?

A: You are not alone. Millions of Americans have chronic or occasional low-back pain. It is difficult to deal with once it occurs, so prevention is very important. Most people with low-back pain have tight hip flexors (muscles that flex the trunk at the hip), tight hamstrings (muscles on the back of the thigh), weak abdominals (you know where those are), and weak lower back extensor muscles (tiny muscles along the spinal cord). To correct these problems, I recommend you do the following exercises every day, and maybe three or four *times* a day. These exercises are taught at the San Francisco Spine Institute or are recommended by the American Academy of Orthopaedic Surgeons.

1. Hamstring stretch. Lie on your back with your knees bent. Loop a long strap under your right foot, holding it with both hands. Keeping your ankle at a right angle, slowly straighten your leg and gently pull it toward you until you feel a stretch in the back of your thigh. Slowly straighten your left leg. Hold 30 seconds. Don't bounce your leg. Work on a slow, even stretch. Repeat several times with each leg. This is an important exercise. Take your time with it.

2. Partial sit-up with half turn. Lie on your back with your knees bent and your right hand behind your head. Begin by contracting your abdominal muscles and pressing your waist into the floor. Then lift your right shoulder and shoulder blade off the floor toward your left knee. Return to the starting position slowly. Repeat, placing your left hand behind your head and lifting your left shoulder toward your right knee. This exercise strengthens your abdominal muscles with emphasis on the muscles that twist your upper body on your lower body (the obliques.).

3. Back leg raises. Lie on your stomach with your forehead supported on a folded towel and arms at your sides. Tighten the muscles in your buttocks and right leg and raise your right leg a few inches from the floor. Hold for a count of 10 and return it to the floor. Repeat five times, taking turns with each leg. This exercise strengthens your lower back muscles. It is probably best not to do this exercise during a period of acute low-back pain. Wait until the pain goes away.

> **Q: I've always wanted to tighten up my waistline but I've never been able to do sit-ups. What am I doing wrong?**

A: We are a nation obsessed with flat stomachs and washboard abs. I often get questions about abdominal exercises. I need to warn you before I get into this, though, there is no such thing as spot reducing. Doing all the sit-ups in the world won't cause you to lose weight around your waist. You will, however, build stronger abs and be able to "hold it all in" better. I don't mean to jest; good abdominal tone and strength is important for good posture, good walking form, and, well, is just plain good for you.

But let's talk about an *abdominal crunch* rather than a sit-up. Sit-ups are old-fashioned, out-of-date, passe, down the road. Get the picture? The new term is abdominal crunch (although I used the term sit-up in the question about low-back pain because that is the term still used in most back clinics and doctor's offices).

If you have never been able to do a sit-up, it is probably because your lower back is arched rather than rounded (although you may not be aware of this). This is due to inflexibility of the lower spine and trying to lift your upper body using a set of tiny muscles called the psoas muscles. Whoa! The psoas muscles are hip flexors and not abdominal muscles at all (although they are located deep within your lower trunk).

Here's how to do an abdominal crunch correctly:

1. Lie on your back with your knees bent (about 90 degrees) and your feet flat on the floor. Place your hands on your thighs.

2. Begin by contracting your abdominals and pushing your spine down into the mat. This rotates the top of your pelvis backward. Check this. You shouldn't be able to slide your fingers under your waist. Are your abdominal muscles tight? Feel them. If all is OK, proceed. Place your hand back on your thigh.

   Now, slowly curl your chin forward as you slide your hands down your thighs until your shoulder blades lift off the floor. Exhale as you curl up. Hold. That's all the movement you need. Feel those abdominals? They are nicely isolated now.

3. S-l-o-w-l-y lower back down as you inhale. Repeat about 10 times. Take as much time curling up as curling down.

If you still have trouble, do this:

Reverse Abdominal Crunch. Begin by sitting up, knees bent to about 90 degrees, chin at your knees, arms reaching out way past your knees. Tuck your chin. Now, curl *DOWN V-E-R-Y* slowly, one vertebra at a time until your back is fully on the mat. This stretches out your lower back muscles and helps you identify the correct muscles to use. You may have to do this several times before trying the abdominal crunch in the usual way again. Get someone to help you by watching to see that *you really do curl-down-one-vertebra-at-a-time*. If a large section of your back tends to come down on the mat all at once, then that is the area you need to work on. Keep at it until you can easily curl one vertebra down at a time and then retry on the regular abdominal crunch. You'll get it, but it may take some time and practice.

> **Q: There's a man in my community who walks with poles. He says this adds to his walking workout. Is he right?**

A: Yes, he is. Walking with poles is a good idea and common in some parts of the country. Walking with poles, especially uphill and downhill, is beneficial for at least three reasons:

1. It lessens the stresses and strains on your lower joints. Walking causes considerable vertical force to travel up your leg from the percussion of the heel at impact with the ground. These impact forces are higher at fast walking speeds and are particularly severe during downhill walking. Walking with poles allows you to absorb some of this force through the poles. For anyone with osteoarthritis or any form of knee, ankle or back problem, considerable advantage is gained by using poles to absorb impact forces by pushing on the ground going uphill and braking the descent going downhill.

2. Walking with poles increases your energy consumption by about 20 to 25%. By transferring some of the force away from the legs and onto the upper-body musculature, you will obtain a better overall workout that shapes and tones your whole body. Now you are improving the fitness of your arms and chest muscles as well as your legs and lungs.

3. Walking with poles improves your balance over uneven terrain, helping to prevent falls. You will particularly notice this in winter and during trail walking.

Here's how to walk with poles. Always walk with two poles. A number of adjustable-length aluminum alloy poles are available at outdoor-sporting goods stores with cork vibration-absorbing grips and rubber bottoms. Some poles even have a spring type of absorption device that prevents jarring of your elbow joints. These poles look like cross-country ski poles but are specialized for walking and hiking. The pole plant is in opposition to the heel strike—that is, you plant the left pole with the right heel strike and vice versa. Start slowly; it's trickier than your think. The last time you thought about how to walk was when you were a toddler.

I started walking with poles while recovering from knee surgery, and now I use them nearly all the time. They definitely increase the intensity of my walk, and I find I can walk farther and longer because they prevent fatigue in my back, legs, and feet.

> **Q: I've been brisk walking for some time now and thoroughly enjoy it. However, I get occasional aches and pains that sometimes persist. How should I treat these ailments?**

A: An acute injury, like the twist of an ankle causing an ankle sprain, sends sharp pains through a body part and requires immediate attention to heal quickly. Acute injuries are usually painful and thus get your attention. These sorts of injuries are rare in walking. But it doesn't sound like that's what you're referring to.

Overuse injuries are common with repetitive movements such as running and jogging because of their high-impact nature. These injuries come on slowly and are the result of repeated stress on a muscle or joint. Overuse injuries often begin with a bothersome little ache or pain and occasionally can become quite debilitating. Overuse injuries with walking are rare, but they can happen. The more out of shape a person is before beginning an exercise program, the more likely an overuse injury will occur (but that doesn't sound like you, either). Because you do not mention a specific ache or pain, I assume you are referring to general sorts of aches and pains—the type for which there appears to be no explanation. If Advil,

Buffered Aspirin, or Tylenol doesn't help, then there may be something more serious. If the same pain persists for several days, you may be looking at an overuse injury.

In general, I recommend that whenever you hurt, use R-I-C-E. Sounds crazy, no? First, **REST.** Don't continue to aggravate the injury. Skip a day or two of walking, or better yet, substitute another activity, such as swimming or cycling, that will allow the sore place to heal. Second, **ICE** the sore area. Use either crushed ice in a sealed baggie or a bag of frozen peas (no, I'm not kidding, it works great!). An ice massage works especially well. Do this by freezing water in a paper or styrofoam cup, peeling back the cup, and then rolling the exposed ice over the sore area repeatedly until the spot is red. Third, if any swelling is present, **COMPRESS** the area with an elastic bandage. Fourth, **ELEVATE** the part to keep swelling down and to encourage venous blood flow for good healing. REST, ICE, COMPRESSION, ELEVATION. It's easy to remember—RICE.

> **Q: I am a very large-breasted woman who has always found exercise to be uncomfortable because my bouncing breasts hurt so much. I also find it embarrassing. What do you suggest?**

A: Many small- and medium-breasted women find it comfortable to walk without a bra, but I recommend that large-breasted women wear one. Breast soreness from excessive movement during sport is due to strain (and possibly microtearing) of connective tissue attachments of the breast to underlying chest muscle. There is no evidence of actual harm to the breast itself, but that doesn't make it less painful. It's no secret that the breasts move not only up and down during movement, but also in outward circular motions (ask any stripper—it's actually easy to get the little twirlies to move in opposing circles). To prevent excessive movement, you want a comfortable bra that will hold your breasts firmly against your chest wall. Look for a bra with the following characteristics:

1. Wide, nonelastic straps designed not to slip off your shoulders during arm movement.
2. A material that is wicking, nonallergenic, and nonabrasive, with a minimum amount of elasticity.
3. Good upward support.
4. Covered fasteners to prevent abrasions.
5. A wide cloth band below the breast to prevent ride up.

Many good sport bras have been on the market for a long time, but most often these are not very comfortable for large-breasted women. Now, Champion Women Action Comfort Strap Sport Top by Champion Jogbra has a good bra in sizes 38/40 C-D to 44/46 D-DD. It features wide, cushioned straps and a Cool-max lining (a type of polypro for wicking sweat away). The Title Nine Sports mail-order catalog shows several sport bras in sizes D/DD (call 800-609-0092).

QUESTIONS ABOUT BODY WEIGHT AND DIETING

We can't seem to get away from this topic because about 48% of American women are on a diet at any one time. And no wonder, for many studies have shown we are a nation of fatties. One highly quoted study published in 1994 revealed that 34% of white American women and 48% of black American women are overweight using a BMI (body mass index) of 27.3 as the definition of overweight. BMI is a ratio of your weight to your height. Here's how to calculate it. Multiply your weight (in pounds) by 703. Divide that by your height (in inches) squared. Recently (June 1998), the National Heart, Lung, and Blood Institute announced a new set of standards in which any adult with a BMI exceeding 25 who is not pregnant, lactating, or a muscular, heavyweight athlete is overweight. That's about 55% of all Americans.

> **Q: How much should I weigh?** (This is a generic question that I get often.)

As implied above, your BMI should not exceed 25. Here's a guideline that you may be more familiar with. Your most desirable weight is within the range of values for your height on the chart below. If you are small boned and sedentary, look at the lower end of the scale. If you are large boned and muscular, you should be somewhere in the middle. At the highest end of the scale, your BMI is 25, and, well, you're getting up there.

Height without shoes	Weight without clothes (pounds)
4'10"	91-119
4'11"	97-124
5'0"	101-128
5'1"	101-132
5'2"	104-137
5'3"	107-141
5'4"	111-146
5'5"	114-150
5'6"	118-155
5'7"	121-160
5'8"	125-164
5'9"	129-169
5'10"	132-174
5'11"	136-179
6'0"	140-184
6'1"	144-189
6'2"	148-195

(Source: World Health Organization)

Q: You haven't emphasized losing weight, and I expected that you would. Doesn't being overweight increase your risk for heart disease?

A: Well, actually, that's a tough question. Most medical scientists state that being overweight or having too much body fat (obesity) increases your risk for heart disease. Others say that there is no evidence that losing weight reduces that risk. In fact, some even claim that losing weight *increases* your risk of heart attack. Not many, however, doubt that being overweight is highly associated with high blood pressure and diabetes—two important risk factors for heart disease in women.

I believe that fatness is not as important as being fit, and data are there to support that belief. Study after study has shown that physical activity and physical fitness are more closely related to risk of heart disease and heart attack than is body weight. For this reason, I've emphasized daily aerobic physical activity, not losing body weight. Over time, if you adhere strictly to the walking program I've outlined and concentrate your food intake on grains, vegetables, and fruits, you will not only improve your fitness but also most likely lose excess body fat and weight.

Q: In Chapter 8 you stated that "dieting" sets us up for failure and that diets don't work. You also said you'd explain that here in FAQs. So why don't diets work?

A: It seems that Americans are always dieting, yet, as a nation, we keep getting fatter. There are several reasons for this. One is that "diets" do not result in desirable lifestyle changes, so we do not learn to eat low-fat, high-fiber foods. Rather, we learn to starve ourselves or to consume foods in crazy combinations (the grapefruit diet, for instance, or the rotation plan) on the theory that they will "burn the fat off." Diets do not teach us anything about the "other side of the story," that what goes in (the calories we consume), must be balanced by what goes out (the calories we expend). Diets make us believe that we can lose weight without increasing our physical activity—a thoroughly flawed concept. The only way to lose body fat and keep it off indefinitely is to be physically active on a regular basis.

But, you say, you lost weight on a diet. Isn't that proof that diets work? My answer is no, it is not. Here's why. If you lost several pounds right away, it wasn't fat; it was water. This is typical of diets high in protein and low in carbohydrates and fats. You can't continue to lose water indefinitely, of course, so the more gradual weight loss that may have followed the initial rapid loss is a combination of fat loss and muscle loss. It is the muscle loss that I am concerned with here. A large part of the total weight lost while on a diet is from your lean body mass—your muscles and vital organs. (Yes, you lose weight from your heart, your kidneys, your liver, etc.) When you decrease caloric intake (i.e., you diet), your body will do the best it can to hold on to some reserve form of energy for an emergency. It goes into a strong conservation mode. We've developed that ability over eons of evolution so that our species didn't die in times of famine. The emergency reserve is your body fat. So while you lose some fat when you are eating fewer calories, you will lose even more muscle. Your body is literally consuming itself. Well, that's fine, isn't it? You're losing weight, right?

No, it isn't at all fine, for two reasons. The first is that while you are losing weight, you are actually getting fatter. That is, the relative proportion of your body that is muscle and organ weight is decreasing *more* than the fat portion. Therefore, as you lose weight, you are actually getting fatter.

FIGURE 10.1
The yo-yo phenomenon

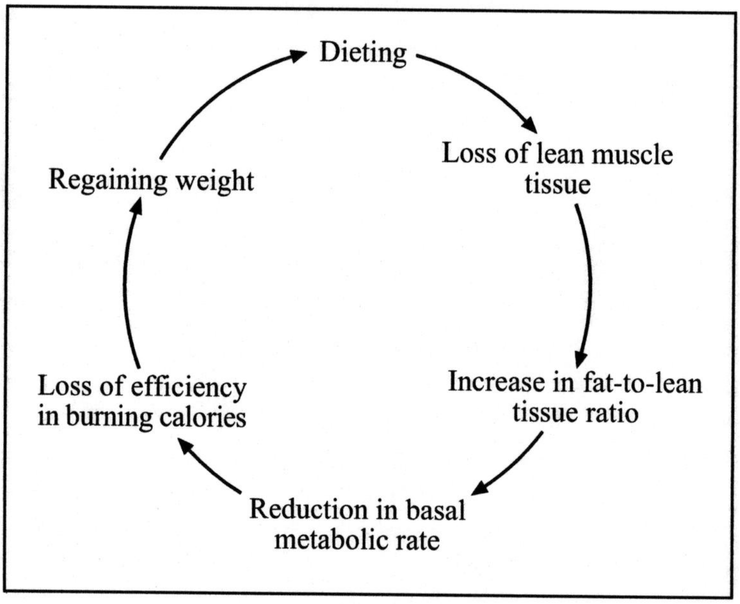

The second reason is that following a diet, you will tend to gain back all that you have lost—and more. Your basal metabolic rate, the rate at which you burn calories to stay alive, depends on the size of your lean body mass—your muscle mass, your organ mass, and your bone mass. The rest of your body—your fat mass—is your reserve energy. Your fat mass draws very little from your basal metabolic rate. So, as your muscle and organ mass decline, so does your basal metabolic rate. Can you see what's going to happen now? You go off the diet, and your body has a lower resting metabolic rate than *before* the diet. When you begin consuming your normal calorie intake again, boom, the weight comes back on because you can't burn calories as well now as before the diet. That's why people not only regain the weight they lost while on a diet but add more.

The medical statistics are astounding. People go on diets, lose a few pounds, regain the weight and add even more. The result is that people who diet frequently end up heavier and fatter. Figure 10.1 illustrates what happens. It's called the yo-yo phenomenon.

QUESTIONS ABOUT FOODS AND DIETARY SUPPLEMENTS

Q: I've heard that vegetarians follow a different food pyramid than the one shown in Chapter 8 (Figure 8.1). Is there a Vegetarian Food Pyramid? And if so, how does it differ from the USDA-approved food pyramid?

A: In November 1997, an organization called Oldways Preservation and Exchange Trust published its new Vegetarian Diet Pyramid. This organization advocates a vegetarian diet and is devoted to the promotion of healthy, environmentally sustainable, and multicultural foods—issues I, too, believe in (and enjoy). So although I am only "almost vegetarian," I thoroughly endorse their new food pyramid, shown in Figure 10.2.

FIGURE 10.2
The healthy traditional vegetarian diet food pyramid

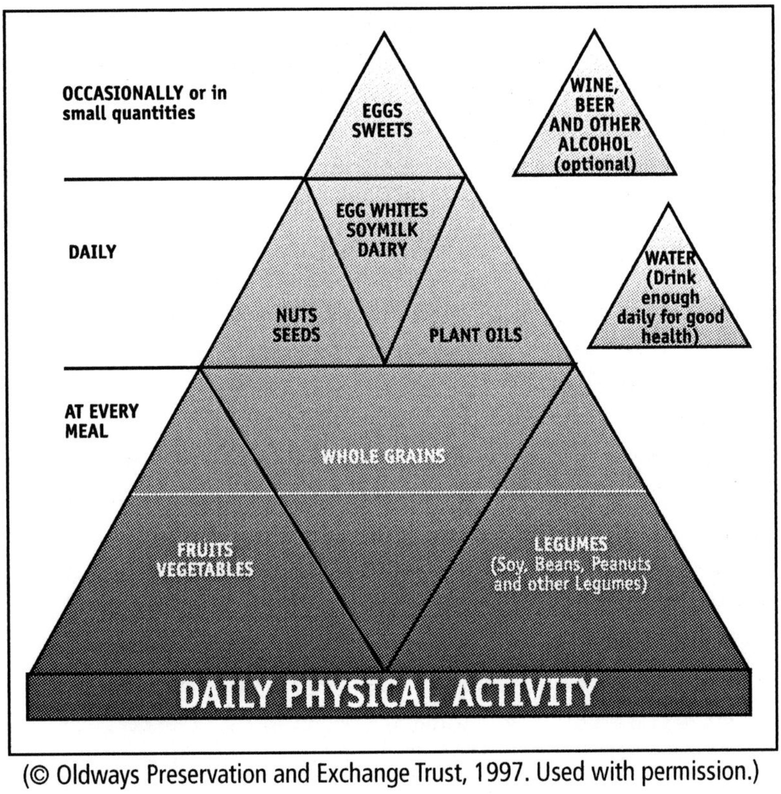

(© Oldways Preservation and Exchange Trust, 1997. Used with permission.)

The USDA Food Pyramid promotes meat, fish, and poultry as the primary sources of protein and only mentions legumes (dried beans and peas) in passing. In Chapter 8, I dealt with this by strongly encouraging you to adopt an almost vegetarian diet by limiting your consumption of animal tissues such as red meat, poultry, and fish to no more than three servings per week, and increasing your consumption of legumes to at least four servings per week.

The Vegetarian Food Pyramid differs by promoting the use of soy, legumes, dairy, nuts, and seeds as primary sources of protein, entirely omitting meat, poultry, and fish. As you can see from Figure 10.1, the base of the pyramid is Daily Physical Activity—no wonder I like this pyramid, eh? Right on! It urges that fruits, vegetables, whole grains, and legumes (soy, beans, peanuts, and other legumes) be eaten *at every meal,* and places egg whites, soymilk, nuts, seeds, and plant oils on the second tier. Whole eggs and sweets are to be consumed "occasionally or in small quantities." There are no recommendations for serving size as in the USDA pyramid. The Vegetarian Food Pyramid represents a very Heart Healthy way to eat, and I strongly endorse it.

> **Q: What's the story on protein if you eat a vegetarian diet? If I adopt an "almost vegetarian" diet, how can I be assured I'll get enough protein?**

A: Americans have long been known to consume too much protein. Most of us, including many vegetarians, eat twice to three times the amount of protein we need. Many scientists believe that is one reason we have so much kidney disease (the digestion of protein places a high acid load on our kidneys) and osteoporosis (high protein consumption leaches calcium from our bones). So, to begin with, we do not need huge quantities of protein to be healthy, as many people believe.

If you are not pregnant or lactating, you can determine your protein needs by multiplying your weight in pounds by 0.36 to get the number of grams of protein you should consume each day. That's not really much protein at all, and only 20% of that needs to be "complete" protein (see next FAQ).

Eating a wide variety of foods on a daily basis—such as dairy products, soy products, legumes, egg whites, grains and vegetables—will readily assure you of sufficient protein without the consumption of meat, poultry and fish. I bet you didn't know that vegetables are a major source of protein for us: 49% of the calories in spinach are from protein, broccoli 47%, lettuce 34%, tomatoes 18%, peanuts 18%, tofu 43%. We need only 10-12% of our total calories from protein, and very few vegetables contain less than 10% protein. So vegetarians need not worry about getting enough protein.

Q: What's a "complete" or "incomplete" protein? I've heard that people who eat a vegetarian diet do not get complete protein.

A: The old phrases "complete" or "incomplete" protein refers to the *quality* of a protein. The quality of a protein is determined by the proportion of the essential amino acids it contains. There are 22 known amino acids. Your body can only make 13 of them. The remaining nine called *essential* amino acids, must be consumed in your diet. A high-quality, or complete protein is one that contains these amino acids in a proportion similar to that of the average body protein. Animal proteins (meat, poultry, fish, eggs, dairy products) are similar to human proteins; we are, after all, animals. And so, animal proteins are high-quality, or complete, proteins. In general, plant proteins do *not* include some of the essential amino acids, so plant proteins are called incomplete, or lower-quality, proteins. The proteins found in soybeans, tofu, tempeh, spirulina, and quinoa (a Latin American seed), however, are complete proteins nutritionally equivalent to animal proteins.

It was once thought that vegetarians had to "pair foods" that were deficient in one or more of the essential amino acids in the same meal to make a complete protein. Thus, complementary foods were eaten together, such as beans with grains, eggs with vegetables, and so forth. We now know that it is sufficient to eat complementary sources of protein on the same day. Simply eating a wide variety of plant-based foods assures this, and it is not necessary to worry about pairing foods to obtain a sufficient amount of high-quality protein.

Q: I've read in various health magazines that eating foods made from soybeans will reduce high blood cholesterol. Is that true? And, if so, are some soy foods better than others?

A: It is well known that people who eat a lot of soy have lower cholesterol levels than people who consume a lot of animal proteins (and saturated fats). Recent evidence suggests that soy lowers both total cholesterol and LDL without also lowering HDL. Although it is not yet clear how soy works, it is known that soy is loaded with isoflavones, which are phytochemicals that act like weak estrogens. Two phytoestrogens, called genistein and daidzein, don't occur in other foods. These plant estrogens also contribute to heart health by protecting LDL against oxidation (thus preventing atherosclerosis) and may keep platelets from clumping together, slowing clotting time. Obviously, phytoestrogens are good heart-protecting substances.

The best sources of these phytoestrogens are soybeans (look for Bird's Eye's frozen Sweet Beans), tofu, tempeh, soy milk, soy flour, textured vegetable protein, and soy nuts. Unfortunately, the isoflavones are not retained in all soy foods. They are *not* found in soy hot dogs, soy cheeses, or soy sauce (which, incidentally, is loaded with sodium).

> **Q: Everything I've read indicates that vitamin E protects you from heart disease. Should I be taking vitamin E supplements?**

A: I am not a strong advocate of vitamin and mineral supplementation because I strongly believe we can get everything we need from our diets—*if* we eat right. That's the primary reason why I did not suggest vitamin supplements in the development of heart healthy habits. However, having said that, I do recommend that people *at known risk* for heart and vascular disease or who *have been diagnosed* with some form of heart disease regularly take a vitamin E supplement.

The benefits of vitamin E, a strong antioxidant, may be considerable. Of greatest importance here, vitamin E may protect LDL-cholesterol from oxidation. If this is true, then atherosclerotic artery blockage could be reduced quite a bit. Some, but not all, studies have shown that vitamin E supplementation may slow the progression of Alzheimer's disease, may boost immune function, and may reverse fibrocystic breast disease in women. But not all studies have shown preventive results.

Dietary sources of vitamin E include green leafy vegetables and oils, nuts and wheat germ. The problem here is that the doses used in most research studies are far more than can be consumed in food. Use of such high doses makes vitamin E a drug, not merely a nutrient. Fortunately, there are few (but some) side effects from doses as high as 1,000 IU (international units) per day. In addition, there are many forms of vitamin E. Should you take alpha-tocopherol, which is the most common form? Or gamma-tocopherol, which is the natural form not found in synthetic forms? Dr. Andrew Weil (*Self-Healing*, 1996) recommends that women take 400 to 800 IU a day of "mixed natural tocopherols" that contain d-alpha, d-beta, d-gamma, and d-delta forms of vitamin E (and refrigerate after opening). I concur with this dosage for people who have heart disease or are at risk for heart disease. Otherwise, my reading of the scientific literature does not indicate that there is an advantage to taking more than 100 IU per day. Eat more soybeans, nuts, and grains to obtain nature's true form of vitamin E.

Q: Will garlic really lower blood cholesterol? If garlic works, will garlic supplements work as well as raw garlic?

A: Several reputable studies (but not all) have shown that the equivalent of one-half to one whole clove of garlic a day can lower cholesterol as much as 9%. That's a significant reduction, but it doesn't work for everyone. Besides, that's a lot of garlic! Enteric-coated pills, which dissolve in the intestine rather than the stomach, cut odor and may even improve the absorption of allicin, the phytochemical thought to be responsible (but no one knows for sure).

Garlic isn't the only vegetable with possible cholesterol-lowering power. Onions, chives, leeks, and scallions—all allium containing vegetables—seem to reduce the production of cholesterol in the liver.

Garlic may also lower blood pressure and inhibit the clotting of blood. People on blood-thinning drugs, or who consume large doses of vitamin E (which also acts as an anticoagulant) should *not* use garlic on daily basis.

Q: My husband's doctor told him to take one aspirin a day to prevent heart disease. Will this work for me too?

A: One of the first steps in the narrowing of an artery is the clumping together of blood platelets. Various blood thinners reduce the tendency for blood to clot by making the platelets less sticky. Aspirin is well known to have blood thinning properties.

Several major studies have shown that long-term use of aspirin confers benefit in patients with an acute myocardial infarction (MI). Subsequent risk of MI, stroke, and death is significantly reduced in such patients, and so there is little doubt that aspirin therapy is beneficial as secondary prevention of health disease. The question remains, however, about the benefits of aspirin therapy in apparently healthy people. In healthy male physicians, taking an aspirin every other day reduced the incidence of non-fatal MI, but the data on stroke were inconclusive. We are still awaiting the results of a similar trial in women healthcare professionals.

My interpretation of the accumulated data is that benefit may result from daily small doses of aspirin *if* you are at high risk of heart attack. In the meantime, I strongly believe that daily physical activity, consumption of a low-fat and high-fiber diet, and stress relief are the best mechanisms for prevention and reversal of heart disease.

Remember, aspirin is a harsh irritant of the stomach lining and certainly counterproductive if you have ulcers, gastritis, or other GI disorders. I recommend you hold the aspirin until much more data is in, especially data on women.

Q: What is the Mediterranean diet? I've heard that it protects you from heart disease even though it is high in fat. Is that true?

A: The French, Italian, Spanish, and Greek cultures all have lower mortality from heart disease than we do, and yet they are known to eat rich, fatty diets and drink alcohol daily. The key characteristics of the so-called Mediterranean diet are a heavy reliance on foods from plant sources (grains, legumes, vegetables, and fruits), the use of olive oil (a predominantly monounsaturated vegetable oil) as the principal fat, a moderate daily use of wine, daily consumption of small amounts of cheese and yogurt (but very little milk), and relatively infrequent intake of other foods of animal origin, especially red meat.

The heart healthy benefits of the Mediterranean diet have been attributed to several features. Even though total fat consumption is high, the Mediterranean diet contains mostly monounsaturated fat. In terms of blood cholesterol and heart disease risk, a diet high in monounsaturated fat may be at least as desirable as a diet low in total fat. Substituting monounsaturated fat for other fats lowers the "bad" LDL-cholesterol and raises the "good" HDL-cholesterol. It may also lower blood pressure and help to regulate blood glucose. In fact, the American Diabetes Association recently recommended a high-monounsaturated fat diet for diabetics who also have high levels of triglycerides and very-low-density-lipoprotein cholesterol (VLDL) because it improves these heart disease risk factors. But a high-monounsaturated fat diet is not suitable for everyone. Anyone who needs to "watch her weight"—which includes most American women—should probably avoid diets high in any kind of fat. But, the substitution of monounsaturated vegetable oils for other forms of fat (saturated and polyunsaturated fats) is probably a good idea (and was emphasized in Chapter 8). Canola oil is a less expensive alternative to olive oil, which is most often an imported, and consequently, expensive food. Canola oil has less saturated fat than any other oil (less than half that of olive oil).

The Mediterranean diet is also high in garlic and spices. Consuming a clove of garlic a day may reduce blood cholesterol and lower blood pressure. Garlic has at least 15 antioxidant chemicals and is a mood elevator.

Several studies have shown that a glass of red wine with dinner may reduce risk of heart attack by 50%. Red wine (but not white wine) contains resveratrol, a plant estrogen (phytoestrogen) that increases HDL, and antioxidants (from the red grape skin) that may decrease damage to artery walls and lower the tendency for blood to clot. The Mediterranean diet usually includes wine, in moderation, every day.

The primary source of protein in the Mediterranean diet is fish, a source of omega-3 fatty acids and vitamin E that reduce risk of heart disease by thinning the blood and preventing blood clots. Finally, the Mediterranean diet includes lots of fresh vegetables and fruits that contain antioxidants, vitamins, minerals, and fiber. All in all, it is a very healthful diet.

The benefits of a Mediterranean diet have not been established in the United States. The French, Italians, Spanish, and Greeks have some good habits that for the most part are missing in Americans. For one thing, they dine. They take lots of time for their main meal, often surrounded by numerous family and friends. They often take a nap afterward. Many believe that it is the reduction in stress and the camaraderie of spirited discussion and love that accompanies the typical Mediterranean dinner that contributes to good heart health.

> **Q: I've heard that one drink a day at meal time helps prevent heart disease. What's the scoop on this?**

A: Several large population studies (Nurses' Health Study, Physicians' Health Study) have shown that moderate alcohol consumption lowers risk for heart disease and reduces overall mortality by about 10%. There may be several reasons for this. Moderate alcohol consumption raises HDL (the "good" cholesterol) and inhibits blood clots. The risk of a heart attack drops significantly in the 24 hours after you have a drink. In addition, alcohol may increase your response to insulin. Increased sensitivity to insulin means that your pancreas does not need to release so much insulin. Lower blood insulin levels are good for the heart because insulin tends to lower HDL and increase blood pressure and triglycerides—all of which are risk factors for heart disease that are particularly important for women.

But all is *not* good news. Alcohol may boost levels of estrogen, which helps fuel the growth of breast cancer. Several studies report increased risk of breast cancer with even one drink a day. The most recent study indicates that women who consume two to five drinks a day have a 41% higher risk of breast cancer. In this study group, there was a 9% increase in risk of breast cancer with every unit of alcohol consumed.

It's hard to be specific about what you should do if you currently drink. Some studies report that red wine protects you from heart disease. The theory is that the flavonoids in red wine (there are fewer in white wine) slow blood-clotting time and inhibit oxidation of LDL-cholesterol—both preventive of atherosclerosis and heart attack. Dark beer is also rich in flavonoids, the pigmented antioxidant found in fruits, vegetables, and whole grains that is protective against heart disease (and cancer). Other studies indicate that no particular alcoholic beverage is better than another and that the superior drink is simply the one that is consumed with a meal. There may be several reasons for this: (1) people who drink with meals typically consume less alcohol than people who are social drinkers, (2) drinking with meals puts a small amount of alcohol in your blood over a relatively longer period of time than in social drinking, and (3) drinking with a meal may provide the alcohol you need for its anticlotting effects just when you need it most—when digested fats pour into the blood, making it stickier and most likely to clot.

Of course, there are many downsides to alcohol consumption. It is easy to become dependent on alcohol for your sense of well-being and to become physically addicted to it if you use it every day. If you use alcohol regularly, follow Dr. Andrew Weil's recommendation that you give yourself two or three alcohol-free days a week. Alcohol impairs calcium absorption by altering the liver's ability to activate vitamin D, and calcium is sorely needed by women to prevent osteoporosis. It may also aggravate hot flashes, insomnia, and depression, all common problems for postmenopausal women. Drinking on an empty stomach will irritate the inner lining of that organ. You should not use alcohol if you have liver disease, urinary problems (common in postmenopausal women), ulcers, or any nervous or mental disease. Remember, too, that alcohol has calories—calories that can not be stored for later use. Therefore, the calories from the food you eat at the same time you drink will end up stored as fat because your body will immediately use the alcohol calories and store the rest. In addition, alcohol does not mix with certain medications: antihistamines; aspirin or other nonsteroidal anti-inflammatory drugs such as ibuprofen (Advil, Motrin); diclofenac (Voltaren); nitrates (Nitrostat); acetaminophen (Tylenol); and certain painkillers and tranquilizers. It also reduces the effectiveness of several medications commonly used in heart disease—propranolol (Inderal) or metoprolol (Lopressor).

On average, one drink a day (two drinks for men) lowers the overall death rate by 10%, so statistically speaking, the benefit outweighs the risk. But *you* are not a statistic, and so it is not so easy deciding whether to drink or not. If you are at low risk of breast cancer, you probably have little to fear with one drink a day, and perhaps much to gain relative to risk of heart disease. If you are at high risk of breast cancer, you should probably abstain. If you are at high risk of heart disease, one alcoholic drink a day may be protective. But if you do not currently drink, I certainly don't recommend starting.

> **Q:** I keep reading that the fish oils protect us from heart disease, but I dislike fish. Should I consider taking fish oil supplements?

A: Oily fish from cold northern waters contain omega-3-fatty acids known as eicosapentaenic acid (EPA) and docosahexaenoic acid (DHA). Quite a mouthful, eh? These two special fatty acids are known as "fish oils." Fish that contain high amounts of these oils include salmon, sardines, mackerel, and herring. The primary benefits of these omega-3 fatty acids are that they reduce the tendency for blood to clot, thereby reducing the risk of heart attack, and they inhibit inflammation, an important step in the development of atherosclerosis. Research has shown that regularly consuming fish oils lowers the triglyceride level in those with elevated triglycerides. Remember that elevated triglycerides is an important risk factor for heart disease in women. (The same effect does not occur with plant forms of omega-3 fatty acids.) Fish oils also lower blood pressure in those with elevated blood pressure.

Clinical trials on fish oils and heart disease, however, have produced confusing results. In men who had myocardial infarction (Diet and Reinfarction Trial), a 29% decline in all-cause mortality occurred compared with the control group, but there was no association between fish intake and coronary heart disease in the Health Professionals Follow-Up Study or the Physicians' Health Study. So evidence that fish oil consumption protects us from heart disease is mixed at best. According to the American Heart Association, there is insufficient evidence on the benefits of fish oils for heart disease to recommend taking fish oil capsules. Besides that, they often produce a fishy odor and gastrointestinal upset. On the other hand, consuming oily cold-water fish several times a week seems reasonable "since dietary fish oils affect 'a myriad of potentially atherogenic processes.'" (Stone, 1996, p. 2339) So forget about fish oil supplements. Perhaps you simply need to find some additional recipes—savory lemon salmon almandine, for example, or baked garlic-ginger salmon. Yum!

> **Q: Homocysteine seems to be the latest thing in heart disease. Should I insist on being tested for this? Or is this just the latest fad? And what about taking vitamin B-complex to lower homocysteine if it is high?**

A: As explained earlier, homocysteine is an amino acid that is a product of the metabolism of animal protein. And it does *not* appear to be a fad. At elevated levels homocysteine damages artery walls and promotes atherosclerosis. The test for homocysteine costs about $70, and recently Medicare and several private insurers agreed to pay for this test. I highly recommend that you request this test. It will probably be a few years before it is done as routinely as the test for blood cholesterol and lipoproteins, but I'm sure that will happen.

If you are found to have high homocysteine levels, taking folic acid (sometimes called B-9) and vitamin B-6 supplements will lower it. Also helpful is vitamin B-12 (cobalamin), a vitamin that many older people are deficient in.

The vitamin supplement known as B-complex contains eight B vitamins: thiamin (B-1), riboflavin (B-2), niacin (B-3), pyridoxine (B-6), folic acid (also called folate or B-9), cobalamin (B-12), pantothenic acid, and biotin, plus two related compounds, choline and inositol. The B vitamins perform a number of metabolic functions, and if you eat a varied and well-balanced diet you should not be deficient in any of them, except maybe B-12. But if you smoke (heaven forbid!), drink alcohol regularly, use recreational drugs, travel a lot, get sick frequently, or have a stressful life, then a B-complex supplement may be good for you. Capsules or tablets that contain 50 milligrams—a B-50 complex—supply 50 milligrams of each of the B vitamins (less for folate, B-12, and biotin) and should be all you need.

If you have elevated homocysteine, you should definitely take B-6, B-9, and probably B-12. Usually the easiest and least expensive way to do this is to take a B-100 complex, one that contains 100 milligrams of each vitamin except for folic acid (400 micrograms) and B-12 and biotin (100 micrograms each). The B vitamins are water soluble, harmless, and can be taken any time of the day. Your urine may turn bright yellow (from riboflavin), but this will diminish over a few days. You may realize other benefits besides reduction of homocysteine.

> **Q:** I have high cholesterol, hypertension, and an occasionally erratic heart rate. My doctor says I should stop drinking coffee, but I love it, especially in the morning. How important is it that I stop drinking coffee?

A: Coffee, and the caffeine in it, does not cause elevated cholesterol, hypertension, or cardiac arrhythmias, but it sure doesn't help them either, particularly if you are addicted to caffeine. I think any kind of addiction is basically unhealthy, and you don't need to drink loads of it to be addicted. If you are dependent on it—that is, you can't function in the morning without coffee—you are addicted even if you drink only one cup a day. Caffeine constricts arteries, and so caffeine addiction will add unnecessarily to the chronic workload of your heart. In addition, caffeine addiction increases sympathetic tone (remember the fight-or-flight responses described in Chapter 9?) and adrenal activity, all of which increase your risk for cardiac arrhythmias. In fact, any kind of stimulant is bad for cardiac arrhythmia—caffeine, nicotine, cocaine, amphetamine, ephedrine. Caffeine is a strong drug, and coffee is the strongest of all caffeine sources. Dr. Andrew Weil claims that his files are filled with "dramatic cures of long-standing conditions, brought about simply by getting people off coffee." (*Natural Health, Natural Medicine*, p. 141) He further declares that you should eliminate coffee if you have tension headaches, anxiety, insomnia, cardiac arrhythmia, coronary heart disease, elevated cholesterol, elevated blood pressure, or a gastrointestinal or urinary disorder. So you see, caffeine can affect many things.

I recommend that you follow your doctor's advice and get off coffee. It takes three full days to break a caffeine addiction, so choose a time when you have few responsibilities. Remember that cola drinks—including diet colas—and tea and coccoa include caffeine. If you get a throbbing headache (a real sign of caffeine addiction), take plain aspirin, not a form of aspirin that contains caffeine like Anacin or Excedrin (check the label).

There are many enjoyable coffee substitutes (and I don't mean decaffeinated coffee—it has caffeine too, plus other substances that can be irritating to the nervous, cardiovascular, and urinary systems). Grain coffees made from roasted grains such as barley, rye, chicory, or beet roots contain no caffeine and are quite good. Some brands are Cafix, Roma, Decapa, Barley Brew, and Lima Yonnoh. Some grocery stores and most health-food stores carry grain coffees.

Herbal teas make excellent coffee substitutes. I particularly enjoy teas made from ginger root, ginseng, orange-spice (like Constant Comment without the caffeine), and peppermint.

If you have been reading health magazines, you've probably read about the health benefits of green tea. Although it contains some caffeine, this tea is filled with healthful antioxidants and substances called catechins that serve as a tonic, have anticancer and antibacterial effects, and may lower cholesterol. Once you have broken your addiction to caffeine, try green tea in moderation.

> **Q: I'd like to lower my daily salt intake but I do not need to go on a strict salt-free diet because my blood pressure is only slightly elevated. What do you recommend?**

A: You are probably wise to do so. Most Americans consume 6 to 20 grams of salt (NaCl) per day, but we only need 1 to 3 grams. Begin by eliminating hidden salt (remember hidden fat?). Prepared foods (canned or boxed) tend to be loaded with hidden salt. Watch for anything with the word sodium (or Na) in it, such as monosodium glutamate, sodium nitrate, sodium sulfite, disodium inosinate, or disodium guanylate.

Next, avoid foods that are real offenders when it comes to salt—chips and pretzels, crackers (read labels), ham, bacon, smoked or cured meats, processed cheese, a commercial hamburger (about 950 mg), low-fat cottage cheese (one cup, 918 mg), dill pickle (928 mg), canned soups (especially minestrone, 2,033 mg!), and hot dogs (627 mg). Learn to read food labels before you make your choices—and take the time to do it carefully.

A good cookbook with low-salt recipes is the American Heart Association Cookbook. Your library may have it. Check it out!

QUESTIONS ABOUT STRESS AND RELATED TOPICS

Q: The concept of meditation really appeals to me. How can I proceed beyond what has been suggested here?

A: Earlier I mentioned the book *Wherever You Go There You Are* by Jon Kabat-Zinn. Some other books I have found helpful are *Everyday Zen* by Charlotte Joko Beck (HarperCollins, 1989) and *Awakening Loving-Kindness* by Pema Chodron (Shambhala Pocket Classics, 1996), and A *Path with Heart* by Jack Kornfield (Bantam Books, 1993). Look also for a series of Mindfulness Meditation Practice Tapes done by Jon Kabat-Zinn. Write to Stress Reduction Tapes, P.O. Box 547, Lexington, MA 02173.

Q: What about yoga or tai chi? There are classes on these practices in my community. Are they good stress reducers?

A: Both are examples of relaxation through body work. In fact, most stress-reduction techniques are connected in some way with yoga. Its interesting that the work yoga comes from Sanskrit words meaning to unite and make whole, referring to the body, mind, and spirit. There are several forms of yoga. Probably the best for relaxation purposes is hatha yoga.

Tai chi chuan is a slow, graceful movement form that combines a meditative focus with physical movement. There are also several forms of tai chi. It is usually easier to find a yoga teacher than a tai chi instructor, but be persistent. To find a teacher, inquire at martial arts schools or wellness centers.

Q: I've always had trouble with self-esteem and I think that is the basis for my relationship problems. I can't afford expensive counseling or private therapists, do you have any suggestions?

A: Women's support groups can be extremely helpful. There are groups that deal with just about everything—consciousness raising, time management, financial assistance, Alcoholics Anonymous, Alanon, problem solving, assertiveness training, emotional intimacy, single parenting, elder care, eating disorders, breast cancer, journal writing, effective listening, Overeaters Anonymous, Course in Miracles groups. The groups often do more than the topic implies. Social support is important. Some of us need more than others, and some of us need to look far and wide to find it. To find a group that you would be interested in (and can contribute to), check out church programs, your HMO, community wellness programs, your employer's wellness program, the local library, the recreation center, the senior center, and inquire about women's centers or clinics and feminist bookstores.

Some interesting books are available about how to keep a journal and how to work through various sorts of problems through journal writing. Expressive writing enhances mindfulness because it is so engrossing, and it relieves stress because you can use it to work out all sorts of things. If you don't know how to start a journal, begin by writing letters—to fictitious people, to God (see *The Color Purple* by Alice Walker), to a deceased parent or husband, to your best friend or the one you wish you had, to yourself, or to your alter ego. You don't have to send them. It's the writing that is therapeutic and that will ultimately rest your mind.

Common Diagnostic Tests for Heart Disease

If it is suspected (or known) that you have heart disease, you will no doubt encounter some of the diagnostic procedures briefly described below. Your doctor should explain any test he or she believes should be done. Be sure to ask for complete descriptions.

COMMONLY USED HEART TESTS

If you have angina, a suspected cardiac arrhythmia, shortness of breath, fainting or lightheadedess, high blood pressure, or other medical problems that might implicate your heart or cardiovascular system, you will most likely be put through a whole battery of tests. Although these explanations below are not complete (that is beyond the scope of this book), they will at least give you a general idea of what to expect and what the tests measure.

Several diagnostic tests can be used to evaluate a potential cardiac arrhythmia. First you will be asked to provide a medical history, have a physical exam, and then most likely, an *electrocardiogram* or ECG, a recording or "picture" of the electrical activity of your heart from the surface of your body. During an ECG, electrodes are placed near your ankles and wrists, as well as on your chest surrounding your heart.

Arrhythmias, however, can be fleeting. Often an arrhythmia will not occur at the exact few moments that an ECG is taken, and so further testing is necessary to detect them. You may be asked to wear a *Holter monitor*, a device that provides a 24-hour tape recording of your heartbeat. This is far more likely to reveal an occasional arrhythmia than an ECG.

To test the functional action of your heart, you may be given an *echocardiogram*, which is an ultrasonic picture of the structure of your heart while it is moving. You may also be asked to complete a stress test—which is an exercise test to "stress" your heart. These tests are described below.

The Electrocardiogram or ECG

This simple test can be done in a doctor's office, and is the standard test given to just about anyone who complains of anything even remotely suggesting heart disease. The ECG provides "tracings" from various "leads," each of which records electrical impulses from a particular location on your body. The ECG (some call it an EKG from the German word for cardiac) provides information about your heart rate, your heart rhythm, the presence of heart damage, an inadequate blood and oxygen supply, and abnormality of heart structure. For example, if you have chest pain, it will be confirmed that it is angina if you have an electrical pattern called S-T depression, a pattern associated with cardiac ischemia. If you have had a "silent heart attack," the ECG will reveal the location and extent of heart damage because scar tissue transmits electrical impulses differently than healthy, undamaged tissue. Structural abnormalities such as an enlarged heart can also be confirmed with an ECG.

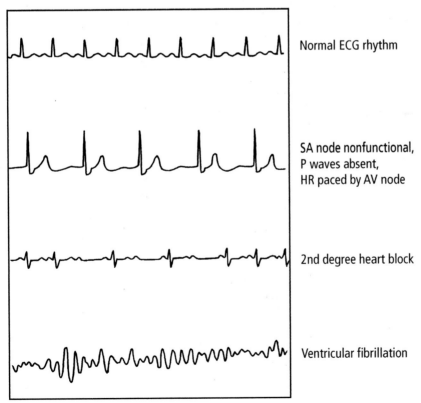

Normal ECG rhythm

SA node nonfunctional,
P waves absent,
HR paced by AV node

2nd degree heart block

Ventricular fibrillation

FIGURE A.1 Normal and abnormal ECG tracings

Unfortunately, an ECG is not always effective in women because it frequently gives false results. Heavy breasts, obesity over the trunk, mitral valve prolapse (common in women) are all things that can skew results. Nevertheless, it is *the* standard test—and it can be quite helpful. If results are "positive," that is, they indicate something is not quite right, or if the results are unclear, you probably will be given either an echocardiogram or a stress test (or both).

The Echocardiogram

This is also a totally non-invasive test meaning it does not intrude on the body. In this case, a microphone-like device called a transducer sends sound waves through your chest (you feel nothing). By changing the location or angle of the transducer, the sound waves bounce off your heart structures (that's the "echo" part). The sonic echoes show how well your heart is pumping blood. It shows the movement of your heart walls and valves, and provides information about the size of your heart, its pumping strength, valve actions, blood flow patterns within your heart, and structural abnormalities. It is the definitive diagnostic test for mitral valve prolapse. It also shows other valve disorders and heart enlargement.

There is a more invasive version of this test, that is particularly useful in women, in which an esophageal transmitter is placed down your throat to get closer to the heart. Of course, this is done under sedation or anesthesia. There is also a form of echocardiogram in which a harmless radio-isotope dye is used (usually thallium). If you have an echocardiogram, ask to see the scans. They are fascinating.

The Stress Test

This is simply an ECG done while you are exercising on a treadmill. The idea here is to "stress" your heart to see what electrical patterns occur. In particular, physicians are looking for arrhythmias and a peculiar electrical pattern called S-T depression which indicates that your heart is experiencing ischemia. The stress test is very helpful because often these conditions occur only when your exert yourself, and consequently, do not show up in your doctor's office. If angina develops or you get especially out-of-breath (remember, you are exercising, this is supposed to happen to a certain extent), then the test is stopped. The test results can be very revealing, but there are often false-positive results in women. That means, the results indicate a problem that isn't really there. And of course, if your test is giving a false-positive result—no one really knows that for sure without giving some other test to verify whether the original result was false or correct after all.

The Stress Thallium Test

This is a stress test—like the one described above—but with a radioisotope dye injected into your veins to "light up" your heart. This is a pretty definitive test. Although not perfect, there are few false-positive results, so if you have an abnormal result, your doctor knows there is definitely something wrong, and will have a pretty good idea of what that is. You are probably wondering "If this test is so great, why don't they just do it in the first place?" Well, most stress tests come out "clean," that is, the results are completely normal and nothing is wrong. Under those circumstances, to skip the other tests and just give a stress thallium test would subject a woman to unnecessary risk (after all, dye has to be injected) and unnecessary expense.

Coronary arteriography

An arteriogram requires *cardiac catheterization*, a procedure in which a tiny plastic tube (a catheter) is inserted into your arm or leg and threaded all the way to your coronary arteries. When the catheter is in place, dye is injected and high speed X-ray photographs record the course of the dye as it flows through your arteries. Pressures within your heart can also be measured. Obstructions and blockages of the coronary arteries are readily seen with this technique, and doctors can tell whether or not you need angioplasty or by-pass surgery (see Appendix B) to open up blood flow to your heart tissues. This test is sometimes called an *angiogram*.

Although this test carries a certain amount of risk, and is expensive, it is considered "the gold standard" of diagnostic tests. It is done in a hospital under sterile conditions in a catheterization laboratory. A local anesthesia is used, but you are typically conscious enough to watch the whole procedure.

A *cerebral angiogram* is essentially the same thing done in the brain to assess the condition of arteries in the brain. Again, radiopaque dyes are used so that X-ray photographs can be taken to determine if there are blockages, and where they are.

Chest X-ray

The chest X-ray has been around for a long, long time, but is still an important test for the evaluation and screening of cardiovascular disease. When X-rays are passed through the chest wall, the rays penetrate different structures at different rates. Tissues that allow most of the rays through show up as dark structures on the X-ray film. Tissues that are dense block many of the rays, and show up as light structures on the X-ray film. A chest X-ray is used in cardiology to detect engorged pulmonary veins (from heart failure), to assess heart size and shape, and to reveal abnormal calcium deposits on the heart valves, in the lungs, in the coronary arteries (in plaque), and in damaged cardiac tissues.

Blood tests

If it is suspected that you have had a heart attack, your blood will be tested for *cardiac enzymes*. Creatine kinase and lactate dehydrogenase levels are elevated within about 24-hours after a heart attack. These enzymes leak into the blood from damaged heart cells, and show whether or not irreversible damage has occurred to heart cells.

Your blood may also be tested for its oxygen level. If your physician wants to know how adequately your heart and lungs are oxygenating your blood, the simplest way is with an infrared oxygen saturation test. In addition, arterial blood may be sampled. This is not a standard blood draw. Sites tested are usually where the pulses can be located: the radial artery in the wrist, the brachial artery in the elbow, or the femoral artery in the groin.

If you are given blood thinning medications to prevent blood clotting, your *prothrombin time* will be measured periodically to determine the effectiveness of the medications. Individual responses differ and correct dosages are important. Prothrombin time determined from a venous blood sample is usually assessed once per month if you are on these medications.

New Diagnostic Techniques

New techniques and devises are being developed that although based on the procedures described above, are much more sophisticated in terms of the resolution of the results. These improvements take the form of better imaging devices and computer-generated digital pictures of the heart in action. One technique, magnetic resonance imaging or MRI, is particularly helpful in identifying damage from a heart attack, diagnosing congenital heart defects, and evaluating disease in the aorta (the huge artery that carries blood from the left ventricle to the rest of the body). Some of these techniques (such as MRI) are non-invasive, and are thus much safer than the older more commonly recognized techniques. Unfortunately, they are expensive and only available in major medical centers.

Common Treatments for Heart Disease

It is beyond the scope of this book to deal extensively with medical treatment. The following information —although brief—is intended to help you understand some of the most common approaches to the treatment of heart disease.

ANGINA

Angina can be treated with drugs that affect the supply of blood to the heart muscle. *Coronary vasodilators* cause blood vessels to relax so that the interior diameter enlarges (dilation). This improves blood flow so more oxygen is brought to heart cells. *Nitroglycerin* is a commonly used drug for angina. It relaxes the veins of the heart as well as the coronary arteries. *Antihypertensive drugs* may also be used to reduce angina. Your blood pressure is the resistance to blood flow that the heart must overcome to pump blood to your body. So blood pressure medications reduce the work that the heart must do. This lowers the need of the heart for oxygen.

CONGESTIVE HEART FAILURE

Various drugs are used to treat congestive heart failure. *Diuretics* eliminate excess water from the blood and body by increasing urination. *Digitalis* increases the pumping action of the heart by strengthening its contraction. Various medications to regulate arterial and/or pulmonary blood pressure may be given. If infection is the source of the problem then antibiotics may be used. Sometimes anti-inflammatory drugs may be necessary. *Vasodilators* expand blood vessels and decrease resistance to blood flow allowing the heart to work more easily. Sometimes surgery is needed to correct heart valve damage, or even to transplant an entirely new heart.

SUDDEN CARDIAC DEATH/CARDIAC ARREST

Cardiac arrest survivors can be treated to prevent future arrests with anti-arrhythmic medications, with surgical procedures that destroy cells that disrupt normal electrical function, or with implanted pacemaker or defibrillator devices that regulate the heart rate and prevent tachycardia and fibrillation.

PERIPHERAL VASCULAR DISEASE

Treatment usually consists of walking—yes! even though exertion causes pain. Regular walking will usually increase ability to walk, climb stairs, and complete other tasks of daily living. Regular walking promotes the development of collateral circulation (a parallel blood supply) in the affected muscles. Medications may be used to thin the blood making it easier for blood to move through the narrowed vessels. In stubborn cases, balloon angioplasty (see below) or peripheral artery by-pass surgery may be necessary to improve blood flow to ischemic tissues.

CARDIAC ARRHYTHMIAS

Supraventricular Tachycardia/Atrial Flutter

Several medications are available that stop this racing of the heart. A surgical procedure known as *catheter ablation* can be used to cauterize the tiny bit of tissue that is causing this very fast rhythm.

Ventricular Tachycardia

The most effective treatment in patients with recurrent ventricular tachycardia is to surgically implant a device called an implantable defibrillator. These devices, now no bigger than a pack of cards, monitor the heart beat, detect arrhythmias, and deliver an internal shock to restore normal heart rhythm (defibrillation). Pretty tricky, huh?

Fibrillation

Implantable defibrillators allow long-term survival of victims of ventricular fibrillation.

Bradycardia/Heart Block/Cardiac Arrest

This is typically treated by implanting a cardiac pacemaker in the chest wall, a device about the size of a silver dollar. A pacemaker stimulates, steadies, or reestablishes a normal heart rhythm.

EMERGENCY CARDIAC CARE

When a person has a heart attack, heart muscle doesn't die immediately, but the damage increases the longer blood flow is blocked. An emergency room procedure called *reperfusion therapy* can sometimes be performed to dissolve a blood clot in a coronary artery and restore blood flow. It is best performed within one to three hours of a heart attack. Therefore, the importance of time to a heart attack victim can't be overemphasized. The procedure involves an intravenous administration of a thrombolytic (clot-dissolving) drug, such as streptokinase or tissue plasminogen activator. The sooner it is done, the more effective it is likely to be.

In the weeks following a heart attack, the extent of heart damage will become clear from the results of some of the diagnostic tests described in Appendix A. When heart tissue dies it can not be restored, but cardiac function can sometimes be restored to tissues with decreased blood flow with the following invasive treatment procedures.

INVASIVE TREATMENT PROCEDURES FOR CORONARY HEART DISEASE

Two procedures have been extremely successful and consequently received a lot of media exposure, so I'm sure you've heard of them both: angioplasty and coronary by-pass surgery. These phases have become a regular part of American cocktail party conversation.

Percutaneous Transluminal Coronary Angioplasty (PTCA)

That's quite a mouthful isn't it. This procedure, called balloon angioplasty or *angioplasty* for short, is designed to widen narrowed coronary arteries so that blood can more adequately flow through heart tissues. It is a lot like coronary arteriography (see Appendix A). It is performed in a catheterization laboratory under sterile conditions and local anesthesia. In this case, however, once the catheter is in place, a second, smaller catheter with a balloon (deflated) on its tip is passed through the first catheter. When the second catheter reaches the narrowed part of the artery, the balloon is inflated. The force exerted by the balloon compresses the fatty plaque and enlarges the interior diameter of the coronary vessel. Then, the balloon is deflated and withdrawn. If the procedure is successful, it results in improved blood flow to heart tissue.

In about 25% of cases, the dilated part of the vessel will become narrow again (restenosis) within the first six months. When this happens, the procedure may be repeated or the physician may decide that coronary by-pass surgery is a better alternative.

Two similar procedures accomplish the same end result. One is *laser angioplasty* in which a laser beam vaporizes or burns away the obstructing plaque. Another is *coronary atherectomy*, in which a cutting device reams or shears the plaque away from the arterial wall. Sometimes these procedures are called debulking. Cutting plaque can damage the artery wall and so extreme care is required.

Coronary Stents

Stenting is a relatively new procedure that involves the insertion of an expandable, metallic, scaffolding device into an artery to prop it open. Usually the artery is opened with a balloon prior to insertion of the stent. Its chief benefit is that restenosis (the artery narrowing again) is unlikely to occur.

Figure B.1 Balloon Angiography

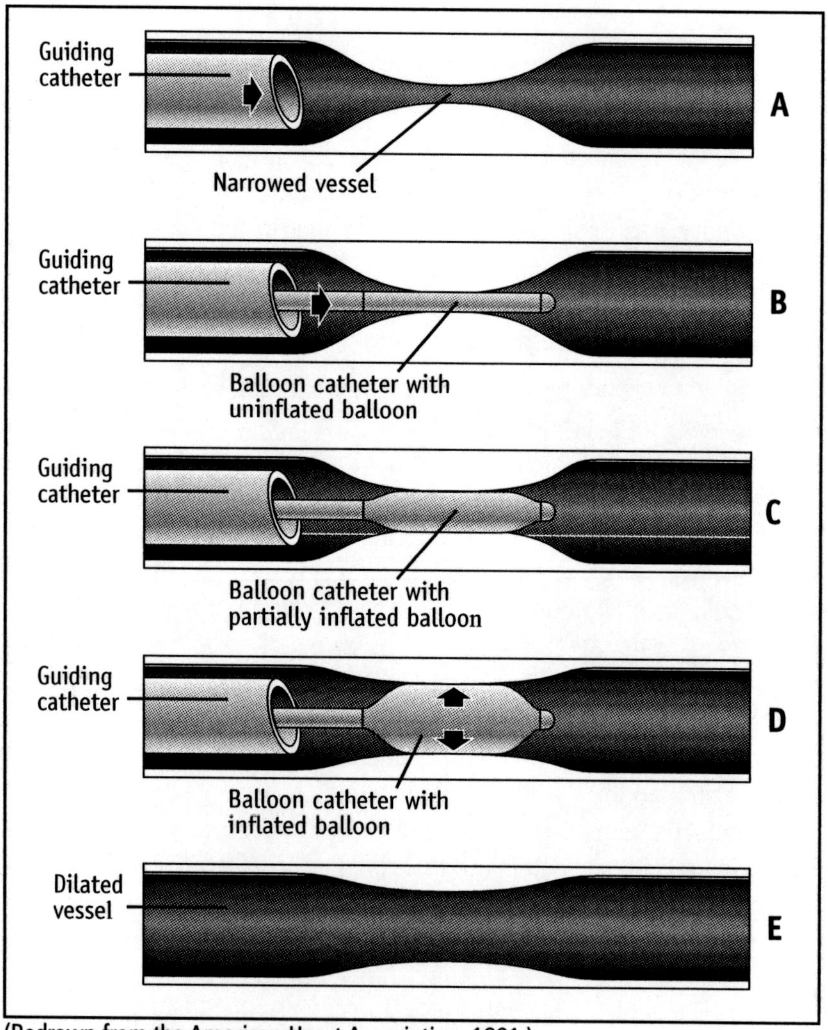

Guiding catheter — **A**

Narrowed vessel

Guiding catheter — **B**

Balloon catheter with uninflated balloon

Guiding catheter — **C**

Balloon catheter with partially inflated balloon

Guiding catheter — **D**

Balloon catheter with inflated balloon

Dilated vessel — **E**

(Redrawn from the American Heart Association, 1991.)

Coronary Artery Bypass Graft Surgery

This procedure is often referred to as open heart surgery. A highly trained surgical specialist removes a blood vessel from another part of the body (usually the leg or inside of the chest wall) and uses it to construct a detour (called a graft) around the blocked part of a coronary artery. One end of the vessel is attached above the blockage, and the other below the blockage. The point is to restore blood flow to the heart muscle. When three such detours are made the patient is said to have "triple by-pass" surgery.

About 300,000 by-pass operations are performed each year in the United States. The surgery substantially improves symptoms in 90% of people who have it done. Of course, none of these procedures do anything to stop the underlying cause of the disease, and new blockages may occur. About 40% of people who have bypass operations have evidence of new blockage within 10 years. This rate may decline, however, as fewer venous and more arterial grafts are done.

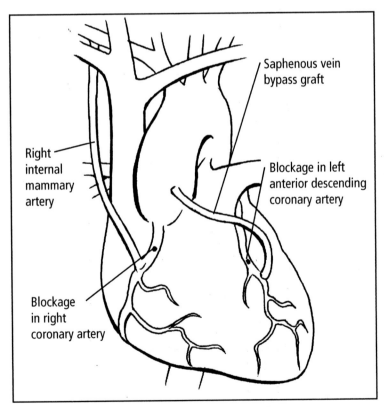

Saphenous vein bypass graft

Right internal mammary artery

Blockage in left anterior descending coronary artery

Blockage in right coronary artery

Figure B.2 Coronary Artery Bypass Surgery
Bypasses around blockage sites can be surgically constructed out of veins taken from the leg (saphenous veins) or from arteries arising near the collarbone (internal mammary arteries).

Heart Transplant

Sometimes the myocardial tissue is so damaged from atherosclerosis, multiple heart attacks, or cardiomyopathy that it essentially dies. This is when the famous "heart-lung machine" comes into use. A mechanical pump removes venous blood from your body, oxygenates it, and pumps it back into your body—during the time just before the heart is removed, and the "new" heart is in place.

There are, of course, myriad problems with heart transplant. First, a compatible tissue match must be found, then there is the traumatic surgery, and then the patient must be "immuno-suppressed" so as not to "reject" the foreign heart. The one-year survival rate of the leading heart transplant centers is now about 80%, but patients commonly live an additional 10 years. Artificial hearts, although they have received a lot of press, have not been successful except as a stopgap measure. It seems there is no beating nature.

DRUG THERAPY TO LOWER HIGH BLOOD PRESSURE

There are many medications to reduce hypertension, but they do not always work. Physicians usually try one medication after another—not randomly, there is a general plan—beginning with *diuretics* to rid the body of excess fluids and sodium (salt). This is usually coupled with reduction of salt in the diet—a lifestyle modification. If this is not sufficient, *beta blockers* may be used to reduce the heart rate and the work of the heart. Another class of drugs are *sympathetic nerve inhibitors.* As their name implies, they inhibit the sympathetic nerves which cause the smooth muscle within arterial walls to contract. *Vasodilator drugs* do the same thing, but do so by directly causing the smooth muscles within blood vessel walls to relax. The result of either type of drug is that the arterioles dilate, which reduces the pressure that is exerted by the vessel walls on the blood within.

There are many more drugs that can be used to lower blood pressure (I mentioned in Chapter 3 that the regulation of blood pressure was VERY complicated). *Angiotensin converting enzyme inhibitors* (simply called *ACE inhibitors*) interfere with a chemical that causes the arterioles to constrict, so the arteries relax. *Calcium channel blockers* act to reduce the heart rate and relax the blood vessels. Often several of these drugs are taken together—and they all have side effects. So sometimes a hypertensive medication regimen is quite unpleasant. Unfortunately, many people stop taking their medications because of the side effects not realizing how seriously they are endangering their health by continuing to have high blood pressure.

The lifestyle approach to lowering high blood pressure (as described in Chapter 3) does not result in negative side effects. These include reduction of dietary salt, loss of excess body fat, reduction of alcohol consumption, and daily physical activity.

How to Determine Your Target Heart Rate Zone

To determine your target heart rate zone, you must first estimate your maximum heart rate. This is almost entirely related to age. It is not influenced by gender or level of fitness. Simply subtract your current age from 220.

This method is usually accurate within 10 beats/min.

STEP 1: Estimating your maximum heart rate:

Maximum heart rate = 220 - age (years)
(estimated)

= 220 - _____

= _____ beats/min

Example:

220 - 54 years = 166 beats/min

STEP 2: Calculating the lower level of your target heart rate zone:

Lower level = 0.70 X Maximum heart rate
(70% maximal heart rate)

= 0.70 X _____

= _____ beats/min.

Example: (using maximum heart rate of 54 year old person calculated above)

0.70 X 166 = 116 beats/min.

STEP 3: Calculating the upper level of your target heart rate zone.

Upper level = 0.85 X Maximum heart rate
(85% maximal heart rate)

= 0.85 X _____

= _____ beats/min.

Example: (using maximum heart rate of 54 year old person calculated above)

0.85 X 166 = 141 beats/min.

The target heart rate zone for the 54 year old person in the example is 116 to 141 beats/min.

Measuring Your Heart Rate

Your heart rate can be determined by counting the number of times your heart contracts in a given period (we will use 10 seconds), and then converting that to beats per minute.

You may take your pulse at your wrist over the radial artery, or on the side of your neck over the carotid artery. Be sure that you press just firmly enough to feel the pulse. If you press too hard, you can interfere with the rhythm.

Wrist:

Using your right hand, place the flat part of your index and middle finger tips on your left wrist near the base of your thumb. When you feel a distinct pulse, count the beats for 10 seconds. Be sure to use a watch with a sweep second hand (don't guess about the 10 seconds).

Neck:

Using your right hand, place the flat part of your index and middle finger tips on the right-front side of your neck just below your jaw (along the side of where your Adam's apple would be). If you are in the correct position, you will not obscure your breathing in any way. It is usually very easy to find this pulse when you have been exercising. When you feel a distinct pulse, count the beats for 10 seconds. Be sure to use a watch with a sweep second hand.

To determine your target 10 second heart rate simply divide your lower level and upper level target heart rates by six.

Example: (using the lower level and upper level target heart rates calculated on p.214-215 for a 54 year old person)

Lower level target heart rate = 116 beats/min

$$\frac{116}{6} = 19 \text{ beats in 10 second}$$

Upper level target heart rate = 141 beats/min

$$\frac{141}{6} = 24 \text{ beats in 10 second}$$

Therefore, a 54 year old person should strive to exercise at an exercise intensity that results in a 10 second heart rate between 19 and 24 beats.

Target Heart Rate Zones and Corresponding 10-Second Heart Rates

This table provides estimated *maximum heart rate* (*MHR*) per minute and corresponding *target heart rate zones* for ages 25 through 85. It also provides 10 second heart rates for the lower and upper levels of the target heart rate zone.

Age	Estimated MHR per minute	70% estimated MHR 60 sec.	70% estimated MHR 10 sec.	85% estimated MHR 60 sec.	85% estimated MHR 10 sec.
25	195	137	23	166	28
30	190	133	22	162	27
35	185	130	22	157	26
40	180	126	21	153	26
45	175	123	21	149	25
50	170	119	20	145	24
55	165	116	19	140	24
60	160	112	19	136	23
65	155	109	18	132	22
70	150	105	18	128	21
75	145	102	17	123	21
80	140	98	16	119	20
85	135	95	15	115	19

Nutrient Profile of Food Groups

FOOD GROUPS	CALORIES	PROTEIN	FAT	FIBER
Grains	68	2	0	high
Vegetables	28	2	0	high
Fruits	40	Tr	0	high
Dairy	89	8	1	none
Meat-Poultry-Fish	177	24	9 high sat. fat	none
Legumes	68	7-10	very low	high
Fats & Oils				
Animal Fats	120	0	30	none
Vegetable Oils	120	0	30	none
Sweets	variable	0	0	none

all values in grams per serving
Tr=trace
Ca=calcium

Vitamins	Minerals	Antioxidants	Phytochemicals	Cholesterol
high	high	high	moderate	none
high	high	high	high	none
high	high	high	high	none
high	high Ca	0	0	high
moderate	Meat is high in iron	0	0	high
high	high	high in selenium	high	0
none	0	Vit. E	0	high
Vit. E	0	Vit. E	0	0
none	0	0	0	0

all values in grams per serving
Tr=trace
Ca=calcium

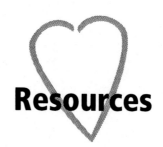

Resources

HEART DISEASE

American Heart Association
7272 Greenville Avenue
Dallas, TX 75231-4596
800-AHA-USA1 or 800-666-7220 (for headquarters)
www.amhrt.org
your city may have a local office, check your phone book

National Heart, Lung and Blood Institute (NHLBI)
Information Center
PO Box 30105
Bethesda, MD 20824-0105
www.nih.gov Once you are into the NIH homepage, go to
"Institutes & Offices" and select NHLBI.

High Blood Pressure Information Center
120/80 National Institutes of Health
Box A.P.
Bethesda, MD 20205

American Medical Association
515 North State Street
Chicago, IL 60610
800-AMA-2350
313-464-5000
www.ama-assn.org

Dean Ornish, MD. *Dr. Dean Ornish's Program for Reversing Heart Disease.*
New York: Ballantine Books, 1990. $15, paper
I highly recommend this book. Part of it is a cookbook.

OBESITY/WEIGHT CONTROL

Bob Greene & Oprah Winfrey. *Make the Connection.* New York: Hyperion,
1996.

Shape Up America Foundation
www.shapeup.org

www.cyberdiet.com

Weight-Control Information Network (WIN)
1 WIN WAY
Bethesda, MD 20892-3665
800-946-8098
301-984-7378
www.niddk.nih.gov/health/nutrit/win.htm

SMOKING/HOW TO QUIT

American Lung Association
1740 Broadway
New York, NY 10019-4374
212-315-8700
800-LUNG-USA
www.lungUSA.org
provides information on quitting smoking

T. Ferguson. *The Smoker's Book of Health.* New York: Putnam, 1987. How
to quite.

DIABETES

American Diabetes Association
1701 North Beauregard St.
Alexandria, VA 22314
800-232-3472
www.diabetes.org

PHYSICAL ACTIVITY AND EXERCISE

American College of Sports Medicine
PO Box 1440
Indianapolis, IN 46206-1440
317-637-9200
www.acsm.org/sportsmed.

Women's Sports Foundation
Eisenhower Park
East Meadow, NY 11554
800-227-3988
www.womenssportsfoundation.com
wosport@aol.com

ACSM Fitness Book. (2nd Edition). Published by the American College of Sports Medicine, 1998. Available from Human Kinetics, Champaign, IL. ISBN 0-88011-783-4.
Programs for improving strength, flexibility, aerobic endurance, and body composition.

Schlosberg, Suzanne & Neporent, Liz. (1996). Fitness for Dummies. Foster City, CA.: IDG Books. (ISBN: I-56884-866-8, $19.99)

Melpomene Institute for Women's Health Research
1010 University Avenue
St. Paul, MN 55104
www.melpomene.org
Publishes a journal several times a year with articles about women's health and physical activity.

Shape Magazine
Weider Publications, Inc.
21100 Erwin Street
Woodland Hills, CA 91367

WALKING

The Rockport Institute
72 Howe Street
Marlboro, MA 01752
A shoe company that specializes in walking shoes. They provide all sorts of information on walking, including clubs and associations in your state.

Prevention Walking Club
Rodale Press
Box 6099
Emmaus, PA 18099
800-441-7761
Quarterly newsletter and annual magazine about walking. $9.97/year.

Walkabout International
835 Fifth Avenue
San Diego, CA 82101
619-231-SHOE

American Volkssport Association
1001 Pat Booker Road
Phoenix Square, Suite 203
University City, TX 78148
512-659-2112
This organization, with regional offices, conducts non-competitive, non-timed walks. They will send you a list of clubs in your state.

US Orienteering Federation
PO Box 1444
Forest Park, GA 30051

The American Institute of Architects
Syndicate Trust Building
919 Olive Street
St. Louis, MO 63101
202-626-7377
Will provide information on architectural walking tours in major US cities

Casey Meyers. *Walking: A Complete Guide to the Complete Exercise.* New York: Random House, 1992.

Therese Iknoian. *Walking Fast.* Champaign, IL: Human Kinetics, 1998. An excellent book.

AUDIO BOOKS (FOR USE DURING WALKING)

Random House Audiobooks
201 East 50th Street
New York, NY 10022

Recorded Books
6306 Aaron Lane
Clinton,MD 20735
800-638-1304

Books on Tape
Box 7900
Newport Beach, CA 92666
800-626-3333

HIKING

Appalachian Mountain Club
5 Joy Street
Boston, MA 02108

Adirondack Mountain Club
172 Ridge Street
Glens Falls, NY 12801

Appalachian Trail Conference
PO Box 807
Harpers Ferry, WV 25425

Colorado Mountain Club
2530 W. Alameda Ave
Denver, CO 80219

Sierra Club
730 Polk Street
San Francisco, CA 94109

American Youth Hostels
1332 I St., NW, Suite 800
Washington, DC 20005

The American Hiking Society
1701 18th Street NW
Washington, DC 20009

WEIGHT LIFTING/WEIGHT TRAINING

Neporent, Liz & Schlosberg, Suzanne. (1997). *Weight Training for Dummies*. Foster City, CA.: IDG Books. (ISBN: 0-7645-5036-5) $19.99.

Fahey, Thomas D. & Hutchinson, Gayle. (1992). *Weight Training for Women*. Mountain View, CA: Mayfield Publishing Company. (ISBN: 1-55934-048-7)

TREADMILL MANUFACTURERS

Aerobics (Pacemaster) 201-256-9700

Cybex: 800-645-5392

Precor: 800-786-8404

Quinton: 800-426-0337

Trotter: 800-677-6544

CROSS-COUNTRY SKI MACHINE MANUFACTURERS

Nordic Track: 800-435-7598

Tunturi: 800-827-8717

STAIR-STEPPER MANUFACTURERS

StairMaster: 800-635-2936

Tunturi: 800-827-8717

Schwinn: 800-SCHWINN

STAIR-CLIMBER MANUFACTURERS

Cybex: 800-645-5392

StairMaster: 800-635-2936

VersaClimber: 800-237-2271

STATIONARY CYCLE MANUFACTURERS

Lifecycle: 800-634-8637

Precor: 800-786-8404

Schwinn: 800-SCHWINN

Tunturi: 800-827-8717

NUTRITION AND DIET

Nutrition Action Healthletter
Center for Science in the Public Interest
1875 Connecticut Avenue, NW, Suite 300
Washington, DC 20009-5728
202-332-9110
www.cspinet.org
You can really trust the information given by this group. An excellent small monthly magazine—$15/year

American Dietetic Association
216 West Jackson Blvd., Suite 800
Chicago, IL 60606
800-366-1655

Tuft's University Diet and Nutrition Letter
PO Box 57857
Boulder, CO 80302-7857
monthly newsletter, $20/year

Vegetarian Times (monthly magazine)
PO Box 420166
Palm Coast, FL 32142-9107
I highly recommend this resource.

COOKBOOKS

Brody, Jane. (1985). *Jane Brody's Good Food Book: Living the High-Carbohydrate Way*. New York: Bantam Books. ($15) A real classic.

Lemlin, Jenne. (1995) *Main-Course Vegetarian Pleasures*. New York: HarperPerennial. ($15)

Messina, M. & Messina, B. (with Ken Setchell). (1994). *The Simple Soybean and Your Health*. Garden City, NY: Avery Publishing Group. A cookbook emphasizing tofu and other soybean products.

Solomon, Jay. (1995). *Lean Bean Cuisine*. Rocklin, CA: Prima Publishing. ($12.95)

Somerville, Annie. (1993). *Fields of Greens: New Vegetarian Recipes from Celebrated Greens Restaurant*. New York: Bantam Books. ($26.95)

Jenkins, Nancy Harmon. (1994). *The Mediterranean Diet Cookbook.* New York: Bantam Books. ($30) A combination cookbook and reference book. One of the best introductions to this region's cuisine. Each recipe comes with a full nutritional analysis.

Sundays at Moosewood Restaurant. (1990). New York: A Fireside Book by Simon & Schuster, Inc. ($16.95)
This is part of a great series of Moosewood cook books.

Ulene, Art & Ward, Mary. (1989). *Count Out Cholesterol Cookbook: American Medical Association Campaign Against Cholesterol.* New York: Feeling Fine (Alfred A. Knopf, Inc.). ($17.95)

The following 5 books are available from Vegetarian Times by Mail, PO Box 921, North Adams, MA 01247-0921:

The New Laurel's Kitchen. $29.95

Tofu Quick & Easy. $8.95

Vegetarian Times Complete Cookbook. $19.95

Vegetarian Times Beginner's Guide. $12.95

The New Vegetarian Epicure. $30.

SOY RECIPES AND SOY PRODUCTS

Messina, Mark. (1994). *The Simple Soybean and Your Health.* Wayne, NJ: Avery. An authoritative book by an expert.

Mindell, Earl. (1995). *Earl Mindell's Soy Miracle.* New York: Simon & Schuster. Good information and recipes.

Ornish, Dean. (1996). *Everyday Cooking.* New York: HarperCollins.

Betsy's Tempeh
S&P Farm
14780 Beardslee Road
Perry, MI 48872
517-675-5213
free recipes

White Wave Soy Foods
Boulder, CO 80301
800-488-9283
call to locate nearest vendor

Vitasoy (makers of soy milk)
800-VITASOY
recipes and information for soymilk products

Soy Connection—Health and Nutrition News About Soy
10525 NW Ambassador Drive, Suite 202
Kansas City, MO 64153

STRESS AND RELAXATION AND THE MIND-BODY CONNECTION

Academy of Guided Imagery
PO Box 2070
Mill Valley, CA 94942
800-726-2070
Publishes a directory of trained imagery practitioners

Domar, Alice & Dreher, Henry. (1996). *Healing Mind, Healthy Women: Using the Mind-Body Connection to Manage Stress and Take Control of Your Health*. New York: Holt.
How to apply principles of the mind-body connection for your health.

Mind/Body Medical Institute
Deaconess Hospital
1 Deaconess Road
Boston, MA 02215
A good source for relaxation tapes.

MEDITATION

Benson, Herbert. (1975). *The Relaxation Response*. New York: Avon. A classic book. Still relevant. Teaches a very simple technique.

Kabat-Zinn, Jon. (1994). *Wherever You Go There You Are*. New York: Hyperion, 1994. My favorite book on mindfulness meditation.

Beck, Charlotte Joko. (1989). *Everyday Zen: Love & Work*. San Francisco: Harper, 1989. A wonderful book on zen meditation.

Chodron, Pema. (1996). Awakening Loving-Kindness. Boston: Shambhala Pocket Classics. A really simple book to understand.

Maharishi International University
1000 N. Fourth Street
Fairfield, IA 52556
515-472-5031
Provides information about local teachers of Transcendental Meditation

LIFESTYLE CHANGE

American Association for Marital and Family Therapist
1100 17 Street NW, 10th Floor
Washington, DC 20036
800-374-2638
Provides list of certified marital or family therapists in your area

American Association of Sex Educators, Counselors and Therapists
435 N. Michigan Avenue, Suite 1717
Chicago, IL 60611
312-644-0828
Referral service that will help you find a reputable sex therapist

American Psychological Association
750 First Street NE
Washington, DC 2002-4242
202-336-5500
Publishes pamphlets on various topics, for example, "Choosing a Psycho-
therapist."

National Mental Health Association
Information Center
1021 Prince Street
Alexandria, VA 22314-2971
703-684-7722
800-969-6642
Provides referrals, support, and information

Self-Help Clearinghouse
St. Clares-Riverside Medical Center
25 Pocono Road
Denville, NY 07834
Has information about support groups on various illnesses.

GENERAL HEALTH INFORMATION

Centers for Disease Control and Prevention
National Center for Chronic Disease Prevention and Health Promotion
MS K-46
4770 Buford Highway, NE
Atlanta, GE 30341
888-232-4674
www.cdc.gov

HEALTH PROMOTION ON THE INTERNET

www.monash.edu.au/health/health.htm

Wellness Web
"The Patient's Network"
www.wellweb.com
Covers both conventional and alternative medicine touching on everything
from cancer to cholesterol to quitting smoking.

Dr. Andrew Weil's *Self Healing* (a monthly newsletter)
42 Pleasant Street
Watertown, MA 02172
617-926-0200
www.drweil.com

Harvard Women's Health Watch
PO Box 420234
Palm Court, FL 32142-0234
A newsletter on women's health issues.

National Women's Health Network
1325 G. Street NW
Washington, D.C. 20005
Has pamphlets on various topics including "Taking Hormones and Women's
Health: Choices, Risks and Benefits."

The Berkeley Wellness Letter
www.enews.com/magazines/ucbwl/

New York Times Women's Health Page
www.Nytimes.com/women/
Nice summaries of women's health issues with a searchable index.

OSTEOPOROSIS

National Osteoporosis Foundation
1150 17th Street, Suite 300
Washington, D.C. 20036-4603
202-223-2226
www.nof.org

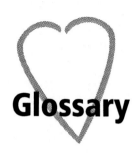

Glossary

Acute - sudden, sharp, of short course.

Acute stress - the term used in this book to indicate the fight-or-flight response to sudden stress (fright, danger, etc.) stimulated by the sympathetic nervous system.

Aerobic - means oxygen requiring. An aerobic metabolic process is one that requires oxygen, can be continued for a long period of time, and is not fatigue producing. Aerobic exercise refers to low-to-moderate intensity exercise that is completed with aerobic metabolic processes. An aerobic exercise is one that is continuous in nature (10 minutes or more), utilizes major muscle groups, and is not exhausting. Walking is considered an aerobic exercise.

Anaerobic - not oxygen requiring. An anaerobic metabolic process is one that does not require oxygen, produces a high rate of energy production, but can be continued for only a limited period of time because it is fatigue producing. Anaerobic exercise is characterized by swift, powerful muscular movements that are fatiguing in nature. Weight lifting is an anaerobic exercise. So is sprint running.

Aneurysm - a ballooning-out of the wall of a vein, artery or heart wall due to the weakening of the wall.

Angina or angina pectoris - chest pain due to coronary heart disease. Occurs when cardiac tissue is deprived of oxygen (ischemia) because the blood supply is blocked or severely reduced.

Angioplasty - also called balloon angioplasty. See *percutaneous transluminal coronary angioplasty*.

Angiotensin converting enzyme inhibitors (ACE inhibitors) - drugs that interfere with a chemical that causes the arterioles to constrict. The result is that the arteries relax. Used in the treatment of hypertension.

Antihypertensive drugs - an entire family of medications that reduce blood pressure.

Antioxidant - substances that inhibit oxidative damage to cells caused by *free radicals*. Antioxidants protect against heart disease, cancer, arthritis, cataracts, and other degenerative conditions. Examples include vitamin A, beta carotene, vitamin C, vitamin E, and the mineral selenium.

Arrhythmia - abnormal rhythm of the heart, irregular heart beats.

Arteriosclerosis - see *atherosclerosis*.

Atherogenic - causing, initiating, or enhancing the development of atherosclerosis, as in a diet high in saturated fat and cholesterol.

Atherosclerosis - from the Greek words *ather* meaning "gruel" or "paste" and sclerosis meaning "hardness." A slow process in which the inner layers of artery walls become thickened and hardened due to the build-up of "plaque." The vessels are narrowed and the flow of blood is reduced. Sometimes called *arteriosclerosis*.

Atrial fibrillation - a very rapid and totally uncoordinated contraction of atrial muscle fibers. See *fibrillation*.

Atrial flutter - a common form of arrhythmia in which the contractions of the atrium exceed the contractions of the venticle. Signifies very inefficient heart action.

Atrophy - the thinning or wasting away of a tissue.

Beta blockers - drugs used to slow the heart rate, relax the blood vessels and lower blood pressure, and reduce the work of the heart.

Blood platelets - see *platelets*.

Blood vessel disease - a form of cardiovascular disease that affects the blood vessels such as hypertension, atherosclerosis, peripheral vascular disease.

Blood lipid profile - the report of your cholesterol and blood lipids (fat) levels. See *cholesterol* and *lipoprotein*.

Body fat distribution - refers to the distribution of body fat on either the upper body (truncal or central) or lower body (gluteal-femoral). Body fat distribution can be determined with *Waist-Hip-Ratio*.

Body Mass Index (BMI) - a means of expressing body weight relative to height. Originally devised for the metric system, it is calculated by dividing body weight in kilograms by the square of height in meters (kg/M^2). Using the English system, it is body weight in pounds times 703, divided by the square of height in inches.

Bradycardia - a very slow resting heart rate, i.e., less than 60 beats per minute.

Bypass surgery - see *coronary artery bypass graft surgery*.

Carbohydrate - the major nutrient, the basic form of dietary energy for your body, a carbohydrate is a compound of carbon, oxygen and hydrogen. One gram of carbohydrate yields 4 kilocalories. A *simple carbohydrate* is readily digested and absorbed for energy. It may also be called a simple sugar or a refined carbohydrate. Examples are table sugar, honey, fructose, molasses, syrup. A *complex carbohydrate* is structurally more complicated and contains vitamins and minerals. Sometimes called *starch*, complex carbohydrates are found in vegetables and grains. Examples are pasta, rice, grains, flour, vegetable matter like potatoes, carrots, etc.

Cardiac arrest - abrupt loss of heart function. Leads to *sudden death*.

Cardiac conductive tissues - the specialized tissues inside the heart that conduct electrochemical impulses making possible a coordinated contraction of the heart. When an ECG is taken, the "recordings" obtained provide information about the health of the cardiac conductive system.

Cardiac enzymes - specific enzymes that are elevated when there has been cardiac tissue damage. These enzymes will be elevated following a heart attack (however mild), and are part of the information gathered by a physician to make an accurate diagnosis of heart attack.

Carotid bruit - an abnormal sound made by the carotid artery when damaged by atherosclerosis. A risk factor for stroke.

Calcium channel blockers - drugs that reduce the heart rate and relax the blood vessels by blocking the uptake of calcium preventing the contraction of muscle tissue. Used in the treatment of hypertension.

Cardiac pacemaker - a very small device implanted in the chest wall that produces electrical impulses that cause the heart to contract in a coordinated and effective manner.

Cardiomyopathy - a viral infection of heart tissue that significantly weakens heart muscle.

Cardiovascular - pertaining to the heart and blood vessels. *Cardio* means heart; *vascular* means blood vessels.

Cardiovascular disease (CVD) - a general term referring to all diseases of the heart and blood vessels.

Cardioversion - application of electric shock to restore a normal heart beat.

Catecholamines - chemical neurotransmitters released from nerve endings that are generally stimulatory in nature. Catecholamines (epinephrine and norepinephrine) increase heart rate and blood pressure, and stimulate breathing.

Cerebral embolism - a blood clot originating elsewhere that lodges in the brain causing a stroke.

Cerebral or subarachnoid hemorrhage - bleeding in the cerebral or subarachnoid (a membrane layer of the brain) area of the brain resulting in stroke.

Cerebral thrombosis - blood clot in the brain resulting in stroke.

Cerebrovascular disease - usually manifested by a stroke, this is similar to coronary heart disease, but occurs in the brain. It describes an impeded blood supply to some part of the brain which may result in injury to that tissue.

Cholesterol - (1) in nutritional terms, cholesterol is a fat-like substance present in animal tissue (meat, fish, poultry, animal fats, egg yolks, whole-milk dairy products). (2) a substance found in blood serum in the form of high-density lipoproteins (HDL-C), low-density lipoproteins (LDL-C), very low-density lipoproteins (VLDL), and chylomicrons. (3) synthesized in the liver, cholesterol is the material from which steroids are produced. The precursor of the sex steroids: estrogen, progesterone, and testosterone. (4) a major component of atherosclerotic plaque, and therefore, having a high level of blood cholesterol is considered a major modifiable risk factor for heart disease and stroke.

Chronic - lasting, enduring, continuous.

Chronic stress - lasting stress that stimulates the stress hormones, particularly the hormones of the adrenal gland. Cortisol is typically elevated with chronic stress. Chronic stress is often regarded as the third (and final) stage of Hans Selye's General Adaptation Syndrome—the Stage of Exhaustion. Chronic stress predisposes people to heart and vascular disease.

Claudication - sometimes called intermittent claudication. Ischemic pain in the legs. See *peripheral vascular disease*.

Congestive heart failure - also called cardiac insufficiency or simply "heart failure." The inability of the heart to pump out all the blood that returns to it. This causes a backup of blood in the veins. Leads to kidney failure, and inability to adequately oxygenate blood in the lungs.

Coronary artery disease (CAD) - same as *coronary heart disease*.

Coronary artery by-pass graft surgery - often referred to as by-pass surgery, or coronary by-pass surgery. A blood vessel (usually a vein) is taken from another part of the body and used to route blood around a narrowed coronary artery so that the heart tissue served by that artery will receive normal blood flow.

Coronary artery spasm - an involuntary contraction of arterial muscle tissue that causes narrowing of the vessel and obstruction of blood flow. Usually occurs suddenly. Thought to be the cause of many *sudden deaths*.

Coronary heart disease (CHD) - often simply called heart disease caused by atherosclerotic narrowing of the coronary arteries.

Coronary occlusion - an obstruction of a coronary artery so that blood does not flow through it. See *coronary thrombosis*.

Coronary thrombosis - the formation of a blood clot in a coronary artery. Also called *coronary occlusion*.

Coronary vasodilators - drugs that cause blood vessels to relax and enlarge in diameter (dilate) so that blood flows more freely.

Cortisol - generally considered the stress hormone, cortisol is released from the adrenal gland in response to chronic stress.

Defibrillation - the use of electric shock paddles to restore normal rhythm in a fibrillating heart.

Dehydration - loss of body fluids, particularly body water (plasma). A potentially dangerous condition.

Descartes' error - refers to the concept of dualism, that the mind and body are totally separate entities (Rene Descartes, a 16th century philosopher).

Diabetes - the inability to utilize glucose (blood sugar) properly. There are three forms: Insulin-dependent diabetes (IDDM; Type I; Juvenile-onset) in which the pancreas fails to produce the required insulin; Noninsulin-dependent diabetes (NIDDM; Type II; Adult-onset) in which the cells become resistant to insulin; and Gestational Diabetes that occurs only during pregnancy.

Diastolic blood pressure - the minimum or lower number in your blood pressure reading as in 120/70.

Dilate, dilation - enlargement of the interior diameter of a blood vessel allowing more blood to flow. Usually occurs as the result of the relaxation of smooth muscle tissue in the wall of the vessel.

Diuretics - drugs used to rid the body of excess fluids.

Diverticulosis - pouches that protrude through weak spots in the colon and fill with digestive wastes.

Dowager's hump - the stooped posture from progressive micro-fracturing of the thoracic spine caused by osteoporosis in old age.

Echocardiogram - an ultrasonic picture of the heart's structure in action. It reveals heart size, shape, and heart wall and heart valve movements.

Electrocardiogram (ECG) - a recording of the electrical activity of the heart obtained from the surface of the body (the wrists, ankles and chest wall). Essential for diagnosis of cardiac arrhythmias and other conditions of the heart.

Endogenous - originating within an organism.

Endometrial hyperplasia - abnormal cellular growth (increase in cell number) of the endometrial lining of the uterus. Considered a risk factor for uterine cancer.

Endometrium - the inner lining of the uterus.

Essential hypertension - hypertension in which the cause is unknown.

Estradiol - the predominant form of endogenous premenopausal estrogen. Estradiol is the most biologically active estrogen.

Estrone - the predominant form of endogenous postmenopausal estrogen. It is secreted by the adrenal glands and is also produced by conversion of adrenal produced androgens (male hormones) by body fat.

Eustress - "appropriate" or positive stress that motivates you to do your best, helps you to meet challenges, inspires you to achieve beyond what you normally would.

Exercise prescription - similar to a medical prescription, but this is a specific description of an exercise program in terms of intensity, frequency, duration and type of exercise (mode) needed to accomplish a precise goal (such as improved cardiovascular fitness or increased strength).

Exogenous - derived from outside the body.

False-positive - a term used for test results that indicate that something is wrong (a *positive* result is bad news) when, in fact, there is nothing wrong.

Fiber - found only in plant foods, fiber is the part of the plant that cannot be digested by the human body. There are two types, *soluble fiber* and *insoluble fiber*. Soluble fiber forms a gel-like material in water, and has been shown to lower blood cholesterol. Insoluble fiber aids elimination of waste in the bowel.

Fibrillation - rapid, uncoordinated contractions of individual heart muscle fibers. This is a totally uncoordinated contraction of heart muscle so that no blood is pumped. A fatal arrhythmia when it occurs in the ventricle. See *ventricular fibrillation* and *defibrillation*.

Fibrin - a protein required for clotting of blood.

Fibrinogen - a soluble blood protein that is converted to fibrin during blood clotting.

Fibrinolysis - the breakdown of fibrin required to dissolve a blood clot

Fight-or-flight response - an almost instant physiological response to stress caused by the sympathetic nervous system that prepares you to fight an enemy or flee for safety. Heart rate increases, blood flow patterns change, blood pressure goes up, blood clots more quickly.

Follicular phase - the phase of the menstrual cycle from just after menses to ovulation. The predominant hormone is estrogen. This phase is characterized by the development of the ovarian follicle and ovum.

Free radical - oxidizing molecules that lack one or more electrons and are therefore unstable compounds. They "steal" electrons from other molecules causing structural atomic damage to cells. *Antioxidants* neutralize them.

General Adaptation Syndrome - a three-stage model originated by Hans Selye in the 1950s. Stage One was the Alarm Reaction, essentially the "fight-or-flight response." Stage Two was the Stage of Resistance in which body functions returned to normal after being aroused in Stage One by a stressor. Stage Three was the Stage of Exhaustion, essentially a state of chronic stress resulting in fatigue and illness.

Glucose - blood sugar, a major source of body fuel. In nutrition, a simple form of sugar that occurs naturally in fruits, and the form in which the starches and complex sugars are converted during digestion.

Glucose intolerance - a glucose tolerance test (GTT) measures the rate at which the cells of the body remove glucose from the blood following the consumption of a sugar solution. A person who is glucose intolerant will not clear the blood of the excess glucose at a normal rate.

Heart murmur - an uncharacteristic heart sound usually of blood shushing past a faulty heart valve.

Hemorrhoids - swollen or dilated veins in the anus or rectum.

Hiatal hernia - the protrusion of a part of the stomach through the opening in the diaphragm for the esophagus. Symptoms include regurgitation of food from the stomach back into the esophagus after eating causing discomfort from the highly acidic stomach fluids.

Hidden fats - fats added to foods in preparation that you don't "see," and may not be aware of. Many "heart healthy foods" are converted to "heart damaging foods" because of hidden fats. Especially in commercially prepared foods. Read food package labels carefully.

High-density lipoprotein-cholesterol (HDL-C) - See *lipoprotein*. HDL-C carries cholesterol to the liver which forms bile acids which are then excreted. Thus, HDL-C is referred to as "good" cholesterol. HDL-C contains a high proportion of protein and a low proportion of lipid (hence high-density).

Homocysteine - an amino acid (a protein building-block). The latest fury of research indicates that this substance, derived from the proteins that we eat (not fat), is the substance that causes microinjury to the inner lining of the arteries, thus initiating the atherosclerotic process.

Hydrogenated - to combine with hydrogen as in to hydrogenate a liquid oil to make margarine.

Hyperglycemia - elevated levels of blood glucose.

Hypoglycemia - low levels of blood glucose.

Hypertension - chronically elevated blood pressure.

Hyperthermia, hyperthermic - pertaining to elevated body temperature due to environmental heat stress or extreme exercise exertion.

Hysterectomy - surgical removal of the uterus (ovary removal, oophorectomy, may sometimes occur as well).

Incidence - an estimate of the new or recurrent cases of a disease or condition. Usually expressed as a rate (per 100,000).

Infective endocarditis - infection of the endocardium, the membrane that lines the chambers of the heart and heart valves.

Insulin - a hormone produced by the pancreas that initiates the cellular uptake of glucose from the blood. Essential for the maintenance of normal blood glucose levels.

Insulin resistance - when cells become resistance to insulin then more than the customary insulin is needed to obtain the same effect. For example, following consumption of a meal, blood glucose increases. The insulin resistant person will require more insulin to lower the blood glucose level than a person who is not insulin resistant.

Insulin sensitivity - essentially the opposite of insulin resistance. This term is used to indicate that insulin resistance has been improved (lessened), i.e., the sensitivity of the cells to insulin is improved, and consequently, the patient is less insulin resistant.

Intima - the innermost, protective epithelial lining of an artery. The surface that is first injured (microdamage) in the beginning process of atherosclerosis.

Invasive - in medicine this word refers to an aggressive or intruding treatment. Surgery is invasive.

Irritable bowel syndrome - thought to be muscle spasms in the bowel and intestinal walls.

Ischemia - inadequate oxygen supply to tissues of the body due to constriction or obstruction of an artery usually causing pain.

Ischemic heart disease - same as coronary heart disease. The term specifically applies to a condition in which there is a decreased oxygen supply to cardiac tissue.

Layering principle - refers to dressing in multiple layers so that air pockets are created to insulate the body.

Lipoprotein - a carrier of cholesterol that is a combination of protein and lipid. See *low-density lipoprotein* and *high-density lipoprotein-cholesterol*.

Lovingkindness - a term referring to the ability to embrace all parts of yourself as well as all parts of the world. The concept originates from Buddhist concepts of love (metta) and compassion (karuna).

Low-density lipoprotein-cholesterol (LDL-C) - See *lipoprotein*. LDL-C is referred to as "bad" cholesterol because it is implicated in the development of atherosclerosis. LDL-C contains a high proportion of triglyceride (fat) and a low proportion of protein (hence, low-density).

Luteal phase - the phase of the menstrual cycle following ovulation. Both estrogen and progesterone are elevated during the luteal phase.

Macrophages - large white blood cells that engulf bacteria and/or damaged cells and cellular debris. They tend to accumulate when there is cell damage.

Menses - menstrual blood flow.

Metabolic syndrome - a group of symptoms known to be a very strong predictor of cardiovascular disease in women. Although the symptoms may be somewhat variable, they appear to be coupled with insulin resistance. The symptoms include low HDL-C, high triglycerides, small and dense LDL-C particles, high cholesterol, hypertension, and upper body obesity.

Mindfulness - being totally aware of the present without judging and without preconception. Intense awareness.

Mitral valve prolapse - a common abnormality (especially in women) of the heart valve between the left atrium (upper chamber) and the left ventricle (lower chamber). The valve protrudes into the atrium during contraction of the ventricle. There is no problem unless the valve leaks and there is regurgitation of blood back into the atrium (mitral valve regurgitation). When this occurs there are symptoms of breathlessness and fatigue.

Monounsaturated fat, or fatty acid - a fatty acid with one unsaturated carbon bond, a single double bond. Dietary monounsaturated fatty acids are thought to be healthful relative to blood cholesterol.

Mortality rate - the actual or estimated number of deaths expressed per 100,000 persons during an interval of time, usually one year.

Murmur - see *Heart murmur*.

Myocardium - the cardiac tissues that contract the heart, literally, heart muscle.

Myocardial infarction (MI) - heart attack. The damage or death of an area of cardiac (heart) tissue resulting from a blocked blood supply to the area.

Myocardial ischemia - occurs when the heart muscle (myocardium) is deprived of an adequate oxygen supply.

Nitroglycerin - a common drug used to subdue *angina*. It relaxes the arteries and veins of the heart allowing blood to flow more readily. This relieves *ischemia*.

Noninsulin-dependent diabetes mellitus (NIDDM) - see *diabetes*.

Obesity - having excess body fat.

Oophorectomy - removal of ovaries. Double oophorectomy often occurs with hysterectomy.

Osteoporosis - a degenerative disease of older age in which there is a severe thinning of bones due to the gradual loss of bone mineral. Osteoporotic bones fracture easily. Particularly common in older women, osteoporosis is manifested by microfractures of the spinal column resulting in dowager's hump, and hip fractures.

Overuse injuries - injuries to the muscles, tendons or joint structures that are common with repetitive movements such as running or jogging.

Overweight - weighing more than 120% of your desirable weight for height or having a Body Mass Index (BMI) greater than 27.3.

Pacemaker - usually an implanted device about the size of a silver dollar that regulates the heart beat at a normal rhythm.

Palpitations - the sensation of an irregular, hard, or pounding feeling in the chest. A common symptom of an arrhythmia.

Parasympathetic nervous system (PNS) - the part of the autonomic (involuntary) nervous system that often counters the sympathetic nervous system.

Perceived exertion - a simple method of rating your exertion. See Chapter 7 section on *Rating of Perceived Exertion*.

Percutaneous transluminal coronary angioplasty - commonly called angioplasty. A procedure used to dilate (widen) narrowed arteries. A catheter with a deflated balloon is passed into the section of artery that is narrowed, the balloon is inflated, and the atherosclerotic material is compressed so that blood will flow more freely.

Peripheral vascular disease - disease in the peripheral (or noncentral) blood vessels of the body. A major symptom is ischemic pain in the legs (claudication) due to atherosclerotic changes in the arteries in the lower extremities.

Phytochemicals - literally means "plant chemicals." Some of these substances are protective from heart disease and cancer (and probably other chronic diseases and conditions also). Several of the most studied phytochemicals are flavones, plant sterols, and allyl sulfides. See Chapter 8, section *What is a Phytochemical?*

Plaque - the deposit of fatty and other substances on the inner linings of artery walls. Characteristic of atherosclerosis.

Platelets, blood - small disc shaped cellular elements in the blood used in clotting. The aggregation of blood platelets is the beginning of the clotting process. The "stickiness" of blood platelets is an important issue in atherosclerosis.

Pleasure/relaxation response - often called the relaxation response (Dr. Herbert Benson), this is the term used in this book to signify the physiological responses stemming from the parasympathetic nervous system that counter the stress response. The heart rate slows, blood pressure is reduced, skin blood flow increases causing a warm feeling, and slow brain waves predominate. This response occurs with meditation.

Premature atrial contractions (PACs) - an extra beat—signified by premature (before it is supposed to occur) electrical activity in the atrium that shows up on an electrocardiogram.

Premature ventricular contractions (PVCs) - an extra beat—signified by premature (before it is supposed to occur) electrical activity in the ventricle that appears on an electrocardiogram. A PVC can often be "felt" by the patient. It feels like an extra beat, a sudden palpitation of the heart.

Prevalence - the number of existing cases. Sometimes expressed as a rate (i.e., *x* number of cases per 100,000).

Proactive - being proactive (as opposed to reactive) means you take responsibility for yourself and that you acknowledge that your behavior is a function of your decisions.

Primary prevention - refers to strategies to prevent the initial development of disease (see *Secondary prevention*).

Progestin - an artificial (made in the laboratory) form of progesterone. An exogenous hormone used in oral contraceptives or in postmenopausal hormone therapy.

Progesterone - an endogenous steroid sex hormone produced during the luteal phase of the menstrual cycle.

Prothrombin time - when blood thinning medications are given, this is a test of blood clotting time.

Reactive - being reactive (as opposed to proactive) means that you do not take responsibility for yourself, and that you do not acknowledge that your behavior is a function of your decisions.

Reperfusion therapy - an emergency procedure performed to dissolve a blood clot in a coronary artery and to restore normal blood flow. To be most effective, it should be performed as soon as possible following a heart attack.

Risk-benefit ratio - pertains to the assessment of risk relative to the assessment of benefit as in the risk-benefit ratio of using postmenopausal hormone therapy.

Risk or risk ratio - the likelihood or probability of death or sustaining a disease or condition as in risk of heart disease.

Saturated fat, or fatty acid - a fatty acid that is thoroughly saturated (or filled) with hydrogen atoms, meaning that every carbon bond has an attached hydrogen atom. The carbon string is fully "hydrogenated." Saturated fatty acids are solid at room temperature, as in animal fat. A diet high in saturated fats should be avoided because it is highly related to elevated blood cholesterol. See *monounsaturated fatty acids, polyunsaturated fatty acids, trans fatty acids.*

Secondary hypertension - hypertension that is dependent or results from another disease, e.g., tumor in the adrenal glands, or a kidney abnormality. The primary problem is not in the vascular system itself.

Secondary prevention - refers to strategies to protect against further spread or worsening of disease. In heart disease the term usually refers to preventing a heart attack, or a second heart attack in someone diagnosed with heart disease.

Selection bias - means that the way subjects were selected for a research study may have affected the results of the study.

Silent ischemia - myocardial ischemia without pain or other symptoms.

Stenosis - a narrowing or constriction of an opening such as a blood vessel or heart valve.

Stress - stress, in the psychological sense, is very difficult to define. In this book it refers to the bodily or emotional responses within a person to some external factor.

Stress incontinence - inability to control leakage of urine with coughing, laughing or exercise.

Stress reactivity - the term used by the American Heart Association for the physical and emotional responses that may negatively affect your heart.

Stress response - the physical and emotional responses to a stressor.

Stress test - usually refers to an exercise test performed on a motor-driven treadmill. The purpose is to "stress" your heart while medical professionals observe the electrical pattern (via *electrocardiogram*) generated by your heart (There are drug tests that may also be referred to as stress tests).

Stressor - anything that causes stress.

Stroke - also called cerebral vascular accident, or apoplexy. A "brain attack" in the same sense we use the phrase "heart attack." Injury to some part of the brain has occurred due to an impeded blood supply.

Sudden death - sudden death occurs unexpectedly and instantaneously or almost immediately after the first onset of symptoms. The most common cause is underlying coronary heart disease.

Supraventricular tachycardia (SVT) - a rhythmic abnormality caused by impulses originating above the ventricles.

Sympathetic nerve inhibitors (antagonists) - drugs used to inhibit the sympathetic nerves that cause the smooth muscle within arterial walls to contract. May be used to reduce blood pressure.

Sympathetic nervous system (SNS) - that part of the autonomic (involuntary) nervous system that is stimulatory in nature. It is the SNS that stimulates the fight-or-flight response.

Systolic pressure - the maximum pressure of blood flow through blood vessels. The upper number in your blood pressure reading as in 120/70.

Tachycardia - an abnormally high heart rate, i.e., 100 beats per minute at rest.

Thrombosis - a blood clot that forms inside a blood vessel or cavity of the heart or brain.

Thrombus - a blood clot.

Trans fatty acid, or trans fat - a hybrid fat created when a liquid unsaturated fatty acid is artificially "hydrogenated" (hydrogen is pumped into it) to make it more solid as in the production of stick margarine. Trans fat has an effect on blood cholesterol that is intermediate between saturated fat and unsaturated fat.

Transient ischemic attack (TIA) - a temporary weakness, clumsiness, loss of feeling, dimness of vision, loss or slurring of speech that is often a warning sign of impending stroke. Symptoms are temporary and there is complete recovery (unlike stroke).

Triglyceride - the most common form of fat found in the body. In the blood, a triglyceride may be contained within high-density lipoprotein, low-density lipoprotein, very low-density lipoprotein, or chylomicron. In the muscle and fat cells, it may be found free (not attached to a carrier substance). Structurally it consists of glycerol plus three (hence the tri-) fatty acids.

Unsaturated fat, or fatty acids - a fatty acid with less than a full complement of hydrogen atoms. When hydrogens are missing, the carbon atoms are bound together as "double bonds." A polyunsaturated fatty acid has several double bonds. Unsaturated fatty acids tend to be liquid, as in vegetable oils. A monounsaturated fatty acid has a single double bond. Dietary poly- and monounsaturated oils are more healthful than are saturated fatty acids.

Urethra - the urinary passage from the bladder to the exterior of the body.

Urethral - pertaining to the urethra.

Values clarification - means defining, examining and perhaps reprioritizing the rules or attitudes you have that guide your life.

Vasodilator drugs - drugs that directly result in the relaxation of smooth muscles in the walls of blood vessels. Used to reduce blood pressure.

Venous thromboembolism - a thromboembolism is a blood clot (thrombosis) that was formed in another part of the body and carried to a lower extremity vein (embolism).

Ventricular fibrillation - see *fibrillation*. A very rapid and totally uncoordinated contraction of ventricular muscle fibers. Usually results in *sudden death*.

Ventricular tachycardia - also called "V-tach." A rapid heart rate that originates in the ventricles. It can be fatal because the efficiency of the heart is so severely reduced.

Waist-hip-ratio (WHR) - a means to assess body fat distribution. Waist circumference is divided by hip circumference.

References

PART I: A WOMAN'S HEART

Chapter 1: De Women Get Heart Disease?

American Heart Association. (1996). *1997 Heart and Stroke Statistical Update*. Dallas, TX.

American Heart Association. (1997). *1998 Heart and Stroke Statistical Update*. Dallas, TX.

American Heart Association. (1997). *Baby Boomers and Cardiovascular Diseases*. Dallas, TX.

American Heart Association. (1997). *Women and Cardiovascular Diseases*. Dallas, TX.

American Heart Association. (1997). *Women, heart disease and stroke statistics*. Dallas, TX.

Anderson, R.N., Kochanek, K.D., & Murphy, S.L. (1997). "Report of final mortality statistics, 1995." *Monthly Vital Statistics Report, 45* (11), suppl. 2. Hyattsville, MD.: National Center for Health Statistics.

"Cardiovascular disease in women: A statement for healthcare professionals from the American Heart Association." *Circulation, 96:* 2468-2482, 1997.

Kavanagh, T. (1992). *Take Heart: A Proven Step-by-Step Program to Improve Your Heart's Health*. Toronto: Key Porter Books, Ltd.

Chapter 2: Understanding Heart Disease

American Heart Association. (1997). *1998 Heart and Stroke Statistical Update*. Dallas, TX.

American Heart Association. (1996). *Heart and Stroke Facts*. Dallas, TX.

Brownson, R.C., Remington, P.L. & Davis, J.R. (Eds.). (1993). *Chronic Disease Epidemiology and Control.* Washington, DC: The American Public Health Association.

Kavanagh, T. (1992). *Take Heart!* Toronto: Key Porter Books.

McGoon, M.D. (Ed.). (1993). *Mayo Clinic Heart Book.* New York: William Morrow and Company, Inc.

Chapter 3: Who is at Risk?

American College of Sports Medicine Position Stand. (1993). "Physical activity, physical fitness and hypertension." *Medicine and Science in Sports and Exercise, 25,* (10), i-x.

American Heart Association. (1996). *Heart and Stroke Facts.* (1996). Dallas, TX.

American Heart Association. (1997). *1998 Heart and Stroke Statistical Update.* Dallas, TX.

Barrett-Connor, E. (1997). "Sex differences in coronary heart disease: Why are women so superior? The 1995 Ancel Keys Lecture." *Circulation, 95,* 252-264.

Brownson, R.C., Remington, P.L., & Davis, J.R., (Eds.) (1993). *Chronic Disease, Epidemiology, and Control.* American Public Health Association, Washington, D.C.

Burt, V.L., Whelton, P., Roccella, E.J., Brown, C., Cutler, J.A., Higgins, M., Horan, M.J., & Labarthe, D. (1995). Prevalence of hypertension in the US adult population. *Hypertension,* 25, 305-313.

"Cigarette Smoking Among Adults—United States, 1993." (1994). *Morbidity and Mortality Weekly Report,* 43(50), 925-929.

Chronic Disease in Minority Populations. (1994). Centers for Disease Control and Prevention, Atlanta, GA.

Duncan, J.J., Gordon, N.F., & Scott, C.B. (1991). "Women walking for health and fitness: how much is enough?" *Journal of the American Medical Association, 266,* 3295-3299.

Kavanagh, T. (1992). *Take Heart!* Toronto: Key Porter Books.

Krummel, D.A. *Cardiovascular Disease.* (1996). In: Krummel, D.A. & P.M. Kris-Etherton (Eds). *Nutrition in Women's Health,* pp. 383-417. Gaithersburg, MD: Aspen Publishers, Inc.

Kuczmarski, R.J., Flegal, K.M., Campbell, S.M., & Johnson, C.L. (1994). "Increasing prevalence of overweight among US adults." *Journal of the American Medical Association, 272* (3), 205-211.

Lokey, E.A., & Tran, Z.V. (1989). "Effects of exercise training on serum lipid and lipoprotein concentration in women: A meta-analysis." *International Journal of Sports Medicine, 10,* 424-429.

McGinnis, J.M., & Foege, W.H. (1993). "Actual causes of death in the United States." *Journal of the American Medical Association,* 270, 2207-2212.

McGoon, M.D. (Ed.) (1993). *Mayo Clinic Heart Book.* New York: William Morrow & Co., Inc.

Mosca, L., Manson, J.E., Sutherland, S.E., Langer, R.D., Manolio, T., Barrett-Connor, E. (1997). "Cardiovascular disease in women: A statement for healthcare professionals from the American Heart Association." *Circulation, 96,* 2468-2482.

Owens, J.F., Matthews, K.A., Wing, R.R., & Kuller, L.H. (1992). "Can physical activity mitigate the effects of aging in middle-age women?" *Circulation, 85,* 1266-1270.

Owens, J.F., Matthews, K.A., Wing, R.R., & Kuller, L.H. (1990). "Physical activity and cardiovascular risk: a cross-sectional study of middle-aged premenopausal women." *Preventive Medicine,* 19, 147-157.

Pagagini-Hill, A., Ross, R.K., & Henderson, B.E. (1988). "Postmenopausal estrogen treatment and stroke: A prospective study." *British Medical Journal, 297,* 519-522.

Pate, R.R., Pratt, M., Blair, S.N., Haskell, W.L. et al. (1995). "Physical activity and public health: A recommendation from the Centers for Disease Control and Prevention and the American College of Sports Medicine." *Journal of the American Medical Association, 273* (5), 402-407.

"Prevalence of selected risk factors for chronic disease by education level in racial/ethnic populations—United States, 1991-1992." (1994). *Morbidity and Mortality Weekly Report, 43* (48), 894-899.

Reaven, P.D., Barrett-Connor, E., & Edelstein, S. (1991). "Relation between leisure-time physical activity and blood pressure in older women." *Circulation, 83,* 559-565.

Sallis, J.F., Haskell, W.L., Fortmann, S.P., Wood, P.D., & Vranizan, K.M. (1986). "Moderate-intensity physical activity and cardiovascular risk factors: The Stanford Five-City Project." *Preventive Medicine, 15,* 561-568.

Semler, T. (1995). All about Eve: The Complete Guide to Women's Health and Well-Being. New York: HarperCollins Publishers.

Sempos, C.T., Cleeman, J.I., Carroll, M.D., Johnson, C.L., Bachorik, P.S., Gordon, D.J., Burt, V.L., Briefel, R.R., Brown, C.D., Lippel, K., & Rifkind, B.M. (1993). "Prevalence of high blood cholesterol among US adults." *Journal of the American Medical Association, 269,* 3009-3014.

Shoenhair, C.L. & Wells, C.L. (1995). "Women, physical activity and coronary heart disease: a review." *Medicine, Exercise, Nutrition, Health, 4,* 200-215.

U.S. Department of Health and Human Services. (1996). *Physical Activity and Health: A Report of the Surgeon General.* Atlanta, GA: US Department of Health and Human Services, Centers for Disease Control and Prevention, National Center for Chronic Disease Prevention and Health Promotion.

Chapter 4: Your Heart Disease Risk Profile

American Heart Association. (1994). *RISKO, a Heart Health Appraisal.* Dallas, TX.

Friedman, M. & Rosenman, R. (1974). *Type A Behavior and Your Health.* Greenwich, CT: Fawcett.

Moser, M. (1992). *Week by Week to a Strong Heart.* New York: Avon Books, pp.129-130.

Nieman, David C. (1996). *Fitness and Sports Medicine: A Health-Related Approach* (3rd Edition). Palo Alto, CA: Bull Publishing Co.

The Preventive and Rehabilitative Cardiac Center at Cedars-Sinai Medical Center, Los Angeles, CA.

VanItallie, T.B. Topography of body fat. In *Anthropometric Standardization Reference Manual,* (pp. 143-149), eds: T.G. Lohman, et al., Champaign, IL: Human Kinetics, 1988.

CHAPTER 5: Estrogen and Heart Disease: What's the Connection?

American Heart Association. (1997). "Cardiovascular disease in women: A statement for healthcare professionals from the American Heart Association." *Circulation, 96,* 2468-2482.

"Effects of estrogen or estrogen/progestin regimens on heart disease risk factors in postmenopausal women: The postmenopausal estrogen/progestin interventions (PEPI) trail." (1995). *Journal of the American Medical Association, 273,* 199-208.

"Effects of hormone replacement therapy on endometrial histology in postmenopausal women: the postmenopausal estrogen/progestin interventions (PEPI) trial." (1996). *Journal of the American Medical Association, 275,* 370-375.

Grady, D., Rubin, S.M., Petitti, D.B., Fox, C.S., Black, D., Ettinger, B., Ernster, V.L., & Cummings, S.R. (1992). "Hormone therapy to prevent disease and prolong life in postmenopausal women." *Annals of Internal Medicine, 117,* 1016-1037.

Grodstein, F., Stampfer, M.J., Manson, J.E., Colditz, G.A., Willett, W.C., Rosner, B., Speizer, F.E., & Hennekens, C.H. (1996). "Postmenopausal estrogen and progestin use and the risk of cardiovascular disease." *New England Journal of Medicine, 335,* 453-461.

Hoh, K.K., Mincemoyer, R., Bui, M.N., Csako, G., Pucino, F., Guetta, V., Waclawiw, M, & Cannon III, R.O. (1997). "Effects of hormone-replacement therapy on fibrinolysis in postmenopausal women." *New England Journal of Medicine, 336,* 683-90.

Knopp, R.H., LaRosa, J.C., & Burkman, R.T. (1993). "Contraception and dyslipidemia." *American Journal of Obstetrics and Gynecology, 168:* 1994-2005.

Krummel, D.A. (1996). Cardiovascular disease. In Krummel, D.A. & Kris-Etherton, P.M., Eds., *Nutrition in Women's Health*, pp. 383-417, Gaithersburg, MD.: Aspen Publications.

Matthews, K.A., Kuller, L.H., Wing, R.R., Meilahn, E.N., & Plantinga, P. (1996). "Prior to use of estrogen replacement therapy, are users healthier than nonusers?" *American Journal of Epidemiology, 143*, 971-978.

Petitti, D.B., Sidney, S., Bernstein, A., Wolf, S., Quesenberry, C., & Ziel, H.K. (1996). "Stroke in users of low-dose oral contraceptives." *New England Journal of Medicine, 335*, 8-15.

Stampfer, M.J., Colditz, G.A., Willett, W.C., Manson, J.E., Rosner, R., Speizer, F.E., & Hennekens, C.H. (1991). "Postmenopausal estrogen therapy and cardiovascular disease: Ten-year follow-up from the Nurses' Health Study." *New England Journal of Medicine, 325*, 756-62.

World Health Organization. *Research on the Menopause in the 1990s.* WHO Technical Report Series #866, Geneva, 1996.

PART II: HEART HEALTHY HABITS.

Chapter 6: Change: Making the Commitment

Covey, Stephen R. (1989). *The Seven Habits of Highly Effective People*. New York: A Fireside Book.

Green, Bob and Oprah Winfrey. (1996). *Making the Connection: Ten Steps to a Better Body and a Better Life*. New York: Hyperion.

Ornstein, R. and Sobel, D. (1989). *Healthy Pleasures*. New York: Addison-Wesley Publishing Co., Inc.

Chapter 7: Exercise: Essential for Your Heart

American College of Sports Medicine. (1996) "Position Stand on Exercise and Fluid Replacement." *Medicine and Science in Sports and Exercise*, 28(1), *i-vii*.

Haskell, W.L. (1995). "Physical activity in the prevention and management of coronary heart disease." *The President's Council on Physical Fitness and Sports Research Digest, Series 2* (1), 1-8.

LaCroix, A.Z., Leveille, S.G., Hecht, J.A., Grothaus, L.C., & Wagner, E.H. (1996). "Does walking decrease the risk of cardiovascular disease hospitalizations and death in older adults?" *Journal of the American Geriatrics Society, 44*, 113-120.

Physical Activity and Cardiovascular Health. (1995). NIH Consensus Statement, December 18-20; 13 (3), 1-33.

Chapter 8: Eating for Your Heart

Brody, J.E. (1985). *Jane Brody's Good Food Book: Living the High-Carbohydrate Way*. New York: Bantam Books.

Dietary Guidelines for Americans. (Fourth Edition). (1995). U.S. Department of Agriculture, U.S. Department of Health and Human Services. Washington, D.C. Home and Garden Bulletin No. 232.

Howard, B.V. & Kritchevsky, D. (1997). "Phytochemicals and cardiovascular disease: A statement for healthcare professionals from the American Heart Association." *Circulation, 95*, 2591-2593.

"New Year's Resolutions: 10 steps to a healthy 1998." *Nutrition Action Healthletter, 25*(1), pp.6-9.

Nutritive Value of Foods. (1986). U.S. Department of Agriculture. Washington, D.C. Home and Garden Bulletin No. 72.

Ornish, D. (1990). *Dr. Dean Ornish's Program for Reversing Heart Disease*. New York: Ballantine Books.

"Phytochemicals: Drugstore in a Salad?" *Consumer Reports on Health*, December, 1995, pp. 133-135.

Step by step: Eating to Lower Your High Blood Cholesterol. (1994). U.S. Department of Health and Human Services, NIH Publication No. 94-2920.

Van Horn, L. (1997). "Fiber, lipids, and coronary heart disease: A statement for healthcare professionals from the Nutrition Committee, American Heart Association." *Circulation*, 95, 2701-82704.

Chapter 9: De-Stressing Your Heart

Benson, Herbert (with Miriam Klipper). (1975). *The Relaxation Response*. New York: Avon.

Benson, Herbert (with Marg Stark). (1996). *Timeless Healing: The Power and Biology of Belief*. New York: Scribner.

Brehm, Barbara A. (1998). *Stress Management: Increasing Your Stress Resistance*. New York: Longman.

Chodron, Pema. (1997). *Awakening Loving-Kindness*. Boston: Shambhala.

Cousins, N. (1989). *Head First: The Biology of Hope*. New York: EP Dutton.

Kabat-Zinn, Jon. (1994). *Wherever You Go There You Are: Mindfulness Meditation in Everyday Life*. New York: Hyperion.

Leonard, George & Michael Murphy. (1995). *The Life We are Given*. New York: A Jeremy P. Tarcher/Putman Book.

Ornish, Dean. (1990). *Dr. Dean Ornish's Program for Reversing Heart Disease*. New York: Ballantine Books.

Ornish, Dean. (1998). *Love & Survival: The Scientific Basis for the Healing Power of Intimacy*. New York: HarperCollins.

Salzberg, Sharon. (1997). *Lovingkindness: The Revolutionary Art of Happiness*. Boston: Shambhala.

Weil, Andrew. (1998). *Dr. Andrew Weil's Self Healing: Creating Natural Health for Your Body and Mind*. May. (a monthly newsletter, call (800)523-3296 to subscribe)

Chapter 10: Frequently Asked Questions (FAQs)

Cook-Fuller, C. (Ed.) (1997). *Nutrition 97/98*. Guilford, CT: Annual Editions, Dushkin/McGraw-Hill, pp. 19- 23; 43-45.

Hennekens, C.H., Dyken, M.L., & Fuster, V. (1997). "Aspirin as a therapeutic agent in cardiovascular disease: A statement for healthcare professionals from the American Heart Association." *Circulation, 96*, 2751-2753.

"Moderate alcohol consumption: New evidence for benefit." (1997) *Harvard Health Letter, 7* (11), 7.

"Six weeks to a healthier back." (1989). *The Physician and Sportsmedicine, 17* (9), 187.

Stone, N. J. (1996). "Fish consumption, fish oil, lipids, and coronary health disease. An AHA Science Advisory." *Circulation, 94*, 2337-2340.

"The Pyramids Go Veg." (1998) *Vegetarian Times*, January, p. 18.

"Uphill & Down: Healthier walking with poles." (1998). *Health + Fitness, Spring Edition, Newsweek*, p. 13.

Weil, Andrew. (1998). *Dr. Andrew Weil's Self-Healing*. (Newsletter) June, p.2.

Weil, Andrew. (1995). *Natural Health, Natural Medicine*. Boston: Houghton Mifflin Company, pp 140-146, 163, 254.

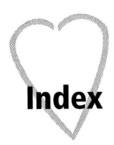

Index

About the Author

Dr. Christine L. Wells is Professor Emeritus of Exercise Science at Arizona State University. She received her Bachelor of Science degree from the University of Michigan, her Master of Science degree from Smith College, and her Ph.D. from the Pennsylvania State University. She completed post-doctoral studies at the University of California at Santa Barbara. She has taught at Dalhousie (Nova Scotia, Canada), Temple University, and Arizona State University.

Dr. Wells has distinguished herself in several areas of study including human temperature regulation, studies of athletic training, and the role of physical activity in fitness and health. She has received numerous awards for her outstanding achievements from The Women's Sports Foundation, Pennsylvania State University, and The American College of Sports Medicine.

She has written extensively in her field and is the author of *Women, Sport and Performance: A Physiological Perspective* (Human Kinetics, 1985, 1991) and *Environment and Human Performance* (with E. Haymes, Human Kinetics, 1986). She recently retired from university teaching to write about women's health issues. She is currently working on a book about menopause. In her spare time, she enjoys cross-country and downhill skiing, mountain hiking, cycling, walking, birding, and her two cats and a dog. She lives in Taos, New Mexico.